MW00620916

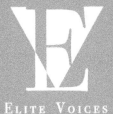

ELITE VOICES

Praise for Rajka

"Delving into ENERGIZED: Feel Fantastic Forever feels like a personal dialogue with Dr. Rajka. Celebrated among her peers as an expert in the field of functional medicine and longevity and echoing the vigor of the Energizer Bunny, Dr. Rajka masterfully integrates her profound insights into the 3-D protocol detailed within. For those aspiring to enhance their health and tap into a world of zest and zeal, this book serves as a guiding light. Embark on this journey and allow Dr. Rajka to lead you towards eternal vitality."

- Betty Murray, PhD, MS, CN, IFMCP

"I would recommend Dr. Rajka, without any reservations, to anyone who is struggling with their health and has not been successful in finding the solution to their problem, or for anyone who is healthy and wants to optimize their overall state of health to perform better in their daily activities and enjoy life to their best abilities.

As a board-certified physician myself, I am very selective in choosing the right health care provider for myself or a loved one. Dr. Rajka is not only an exceptional functional medicine doctor, but she is also a board-certified family physician with many years of experience, and that level of experience gives her an edge above many other practitioners because she has seen a multitude of medically complex cases throughout her career.

She has excellent bedside manners, is very thorough in her history taking and physical examination. She will spend the necessary time to ask all the pertinent questions, including questions that no other doctor has asked before, that are relevant to determine the right diagnosis, and will order extensive laboratory testing if appropriate to your specific case.

My state of health and energy levels have improved significantly since she evaluated me, and I am looking forward to continuing my journey with her for many years to come."

- Pedro Gonzalez, MD

"I cannot overstate how much I appreciate Dr. Rajka's breadth of knowledge and willingness to 'look outside the box' in directing me towards optimal health. Her unique background, exceptional bedside manner, and compassionate care are truly second to none. She works tirelessly with her patients to make them an active participant in their care—the tools I have learned from Dr. Rajka will without a doubt benefit me the rest of my life. She is the first provider I have felt truly heard by —not only an exceptional physician, but an exceptional human being. I would recommend Dr. Rajka without the slightest hesitation to anyone who is struggling to find an effective solution to their symptoms or is simply trying to better their health and quality of life. From the bottom of my heart, THANK YOU, Dr. Rajka and team!"

- Kelsey Yerkes

"Dr. Rajka is simply outstanding!!! Her expertise, approach, and understanding of health matters has helped me beyond the words I can write. She helped me address a number of health matters that came up quickly and caused me some pretty uncomfortable symptoms. She also uncovered several health conditions I had, but didn't know until we ran tests she recommended. Amazingly, these underlying conditions were very significant and probably were the primary causes of what came up for me initially. If it were not for Dr. Rajka, I would have started prescription drugs my family doctor prescribed but were not needed. Also, things I was not aware of would have only gotten worse, and I feel comfortable in saying that I probably would not have found out about them if it was not for Dr. Rajka's diligence. I am so pleased that after many months of her help, I've successfully addressed so many things, and I truly feel better than I have in years. This kind of help is priceless, and my quality of life benefitted greatly. This is a glowing recommendation, and yet I could say more …happy and grateful to be healthier, thank you, Dr. Rajka!!"

- Laurie Urbancik

"I'm very thankful to have found Simply Health Institute & Dr. Rajka after suffering with anxiety! Once I started getting panic attacks, etc., I knew something was going on, and I needed to do something to prioritize my health. After going to my PCP, and telling them how I felt, I was simply told it's okay and given a medication and told to go on my way. I knew I did not want to do that for the rest of my life. It has been about 6 months since I have been working with Dr. Rajka and have improved greatly. She is attentive, organized, and very supportive, and her staff is also great! She focuses on factors that affect your health that most providers miss, or don't even check. Everyone's care is very personalized, and that is the best thing she did for me. Since my care has started, I have referred my husband and my mother, and both have loved it and have had great experiences as well! I will forever be Dr. Rajka's patient! Thank you so much, and I appreciate you guys so much more. I can finally say I have my life back."

- Alexsandra Garcia

ENERGIZED

FEEL **FANTASTIC** FOREVER

ENERGIZED

FEEL **FANTASTIC** FOREVER

Rajka Milanovic Galbraith, MD

ELITE VOICES

ELITE VOICES
San Antonio, TX 78229

First Edition, October 2023
ISBN: 978-1-63765-484-2
Library of Congress Control Number: 2023915976

Our mission is to empower individuals and businesses to enhance their professional brand by becoming recognized experts in their field. We provide the tools and resources to help our clients become authors, establish a strong personal brand, and grow their business to achieve greater visibility, credibility, and financial success.

To Kerry, Liam, and Liv: My everything!

Contents

Foreword

We are living in unusually difficult times. Slowly and insidiously, over 350,000 new chemicals have been introduced into our world, and only 500 have been evaluated carefully for their toxicity to humans. Our exposure to electromagnetic frequencies has grown exponentially, with only token reassurance about how safe this is. Our lives are out-of-control stressful, to which the COVID epidemic has added a level of fear and isolation unknown to previous generations.

It should come as no surprise that within this context, many of us have grown accustomed to a lower level of energy or vitality that we accept as normal, and are content to simply make it through each day. If we compare notes with our family, friends, and neighbors, they are all experiencing the same depletion of vital energies, so who are we to complain?

I have known Rajka professionally for many years, and I am delighted that she has taken the time to distill her many years of clinical and personal experience into this concise volume of information. Here is a relatively simple handbook for how, exactly, to look at your habits and behaviors and decide that perhaps you could make a few changes to feel better. She breaks down her information into several acronyms, and then goes into detail about how to examine your diet, eating habits, sleep habits, stressors, and chemical exposures, to the end of feeling much better.

If you or your loved ones would pick just a few of these suggestions and implement them, I am certain your effort would be well rewarded. Once those have been shown to be of benefit, you will then, on your own, want to add more and more of these suggestions as you watch your health improve.

I would encourage readers to not just skim these pages, but actually study them and make a commitment to change(s). Follow up with the many resources she provides both in this book and online.

There is a wealth of timely information in these pages, and I hope you can take this in and find yourself able to have the energy to live your fullest life with joy and creativity.

To your health and happiness,

Neil Nathan, M.D.

Author of the best-selling *Toxic: Heal Your Body from Mold Toxicity, Lyme Disease, Multiple Chemical Sensitivity, and Chronic Environmental Illness,* and the soon-to-be released *The Sensitive Patient's Healing Guide.*

Introduction

I stepped out onto my balcony and took a sip of coffee. Ah, that first sip of my morning latte, nothing beats it. I gazed out at the most gorgeous view I could ever imagine: the Puget Sound from just above the Mukilteo ferry. The baby-blue early morning sky reflecting off the calm water was a mirror image to the contented calm I felt that morning. As I quickly finished my coffee and drove down the coast to work at my first practice post-residency, I was elated. I had worked my whole life to become a doctor. It had been my childhood dream ever since I was five.

I arrived at the office and began looking through the schedule. I had only been at the practice for a few short months. It was the fall of 1997, and I was one of ten family doctors who were part of Everett Family Practice Center, the longest standing family practice clinic in Everett, Washington.

My first patient of the day was in her late forties. She came in complaining of fatigue. This seemed to be a pretty common complaint. During training, they told us to do an exam, run some labs, and if nothing was abnormal, suggest the patient was depressed. This never sat right with me. But this is what I did. I examined the patient and ordered labs.

When she came back a couple of weeks later and all her labs were normal, I asked if she was possibly depressed. She shook her head, looking defeated, and then got up and exited the room. I followed her out to let her into the lobby, as it was customary to do.

Her girlfriend approached and asked excitedly, "Well? What's wrong with you?"

Clearly upset, my patient replied, "That dumb doctor doesn't know what's wrong with me!"

"Dumb doctor." I wasn't a dumb doctor. I'd spent years training to be a doctor. Putting my ego aside, I was disappointed that these many years of training didn't allow me to give her answers, to give her hope, let alone allow me to make her feel better. I had no answers. And this wasn't the first time this had happened within those few short months of practice.

Little did I know that this fatigue I had seen over and over and over again was something that I was already suffering from, something that would almost lead to my demise.

I knew something was missing. I wasn't really curing anyone. I went into medicine because I wanted to *cure everyone*. I went into medicine because I had envisioned myself being a family doctor, taking care of infants, delivering babies, and doing their exams after they were born. And, soon after, their aunts and uncles would come see me. Even the reluctant fathers, who seemingly were healthy, eventually came in.

I felt on top of the world, but I wasn't *curing* anyone. Had I really reflected on my life to this point, I would have realized that I was pretty darn fatigued myself. During residency, it was an effort to even get out of bed. Mind you, the hours were pretty rough, but not everyone had this problem. On more than one occasion I fell asleep standing up. Yes, we were sleep deprived, but even with a full night's sleep, I just never *ever* felt refreshed. People started to notice. I felt just like the patients who came in with fatigue and had normal labs. My labs were normal too. I didn't want people to think I was depressed because I didn't *feel* depressed. Like me, many of my fatigued patients were not depressed. They were just tired, plain and simple.

I was starting to be labeled as lazy. I would show up just in time to pre-round on my patients so I could present to the resident and the attending. I would often-times sleep through two beepers *and* my cell phone. A lot of my friends started to make fun of me. At least their jests I could stomach. They were my friends. I would poke fun at myself too. I didn't know which was more embarrassing:

falling asleep while on a date (could you imagine my love life then?), or falling asleep at a rock concert.

Yep, I fell asleep at the Rock and Roll Hall of Fame inaugural rock concert on September 2, 1995. I was awake long enough to hear Bruce Springsteen play. The Boss was one of my favorites. In fact, he was one of the first concerts I saw growing up, in high school, without adult supervision. Who falls asleep at a rock concert?!

Post-residency, I spent three months sleeping every second I wasn't working. I didn't have much of a social life. I kept wondering, *Why do I feel so tired?* I ate healthily. While I loved to exercise, I wasn't overexercising. I trained for a couple of big events during residency, including a marathon and a bike tour, which took me from Columbus to Chillicothe and back in only two days. While some of the time I felt okay, a lot of the time I was just plain old tired.

I was so tired by my third year in residency, and it wasn't just the physical stress. It had also become mental and emotional. My dad had a hemorrhagic bleed during my last year in residency. He was only fifty-seven years old. I spent a lot of time driving between Columbus and Cleveland to visit him, first in the ICU, then in the hospital, and then in the rehab facility. Not knowing for weeks if he was going to make it, and not knowing if he would have any quality of life if he did survive. This was the same man who was so proud to watch me walk across the stage and get my medical degree. I was the first doctor in the family.

Six weeks before completing residency, there was one day in which I'd had enough. I marched up to my residency director's office and told him I quit. I took the elevator to the basement of the hospital, down to the abandoned corridor filled with old gurneys. It was still and silent. I put my back against the wall, slid to the floor, and cried and cried and cried, until I had nothing left. I had nothing left to give.

With the steady support of my residency director, the infamous Dr. Scully, I was able to finish out those remaining six weeks and graduate from my family practice residency. I moved to Seattle and took my first job doing what had been my calling since the age of five. What I didn't know was that it would take me over twenty-six years and another entire medical school education in cost to figure out how to truly heal my patients.

Now, after a decade of practicing functional medicine, I've recovered tens of thousands of patients' health and vitality, including my own.

I am writing this book in the hopes of preventing needless suffering.

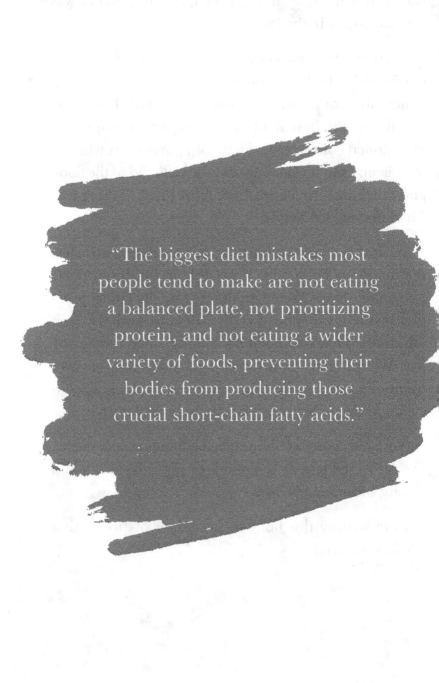

"The biggest diet mistakes most people tend to make are not eating a balanced plate, not prioritizing protein, and not eating a wider variety of foods, preventing their bodies from producing those crucial short-chain fatty acids."

Chapter 1

The First *D*: Diet

I t took me over ten years to create my 3-D Energy Protocol. This protocol delivers results every single time, so that you don't have to spend decades and hundreds of thousands of dollars to reclaim your health. It's why people fly in from all over the world to see me, and why I have been nicknamed the Energizer Bunny and the Go-To Doctor *for* Doctors.

The 3 *D*s:

Diet + Nutrients
Digestion
Detoxification

Through my various programs, both in-office and online, I have crafted the right steps in the right order with the right amount of support. However, as the name 3-D implies, it is multidimensional. The three *D*s are foundational for increasing your energy. Once you've reclaimed your energy, you'll be ready to implement the additional six steps, which consist of three *S*s and three *M*s, but we'll get to that later.

Have you ever wondered why no one can agree on which diet is the actual *best* diet? Is it gluten-free? Dairy-free? Paleo, keto? Atkins, low carb, high carb, low fat? Or is it something else? Which one is it? Because of my love of nutrigenetics—the study of bypassing defective genes with nutrients (vitamins and minerals)—I learned that we are all genetically different, and there is *no* one-size-fits-all diet.

Over the last decade, I developed the T.A.S.K. method to the Abundant Diet 365. Having tried almost every diet on the market, including low fat, low carb, paleo, keto, and even Body for Life and Weight Watchers, I have developed a process by learning my own genetic variations. I was able to learn how to eat for my metabolic makeup. I can now determine how someone needs to eat, without even knowing their genetics, because I have learned how to reverse engineer it. I have also identified several key things that most people get wrong, which keeps them inflamed and does not allow them to lose weight. There is even one area that most functional medicine practitioners get wrong, contributing to the development of unintentional food sensitivities and lots of wasted time.

I've been in the weight loss industry since 1997. Back when I was working 100-plus hours a week, I was also moonlighting in a weight loss clinic. This clinic prescribed a low-calorie diet combined with medications, such as phentermine, fenfluramine, and Prozac, all of which carried side effects—some serious and some even fatal. While many people lost weight, many people also regained it once these medications were stopped. That's where I learned how you *shouldn't* approach weight loss programs. Now I know how to help people lose weight in a safe and easy fashion by doing it the *right* way.

In my late teens, I was particularly stressed. I had a very difficult AP teacher for English. Nobody liked her. In fact, she was so disliked that her house was egged and spray-painted with profanity. It was sad to see, but she did nothing to facilitate a nurturing relationship with her students, including me. No matter how hard I tried, I could get nothing better than a C on the papers I wrote.

Sadly, I could spend all weekend writing a paper, turn it in, and get the same grade: a C! While I wrote these papers, I ate countless pieces of toast smothered in butter and peanut butter. I used food as a crutch whenever I was stressed. Even if I could avoid eating, I was very stress responsive, meaning that when I was stressed, I tended to stay stressed. I had not learned any of the techniques to mitigate stress I now know and teach my patients. Stress causes an increase in cortisol, which makes you inflamed and causes your insulin level to rise. Insulin drops your blood sugar, which causes you to crave carbohydrates, which then causes you to eat more and more carbs. Over time, your insulin doesn't work as well, leading to insulin resistance. Insulin resistance, combined with inflammation, makes losing weight incredibly difficult.

Let's put into perspective the impact stress can have on our body's reaction to eating.

One of my favorite mentors and now friend, JJ Virgin, lost weight during a weeklong meditation retreat, despite eating more than she usually does. One can assume a weeklong meditation retreat would be a rather stress-free environment, right? So when she admitted to losing weight, even though she was eating more than usual, I found this juxtaposition fascinating.

During every stressful time period in my life—including my junior year of high school, the first year of college, the first year of medical school, the first year of residency, and even every single vacation that I ever took—I could easily gain five pounds. Sometimes in as little as a week! I jogged five miles a day while away on vacation. Can you imagine having to jog just to be able to maintain weight so that you can enjoy a *vacation*? That is how stress responsive I was, and how big a role being stressed can play in your life.

I learned that if I started the day with carbohydrates, I would continue to crave food, which resulted in over-eating. If only I had known how to eat a balanced plate, which is what I now teach my patients. I quickly learned that carbs were *not* my friend, so I limited them. This was without even knowing my genetics. As it turns out, I have a doubly mutated AMY1 gene, meaning that my metabolism of starch is potentially 70 percent slower than the average person. I think the worst diet I ever tried was the low-fat, trendy diet of the nineties. You traded fat, which helps you feel satiated and full, for more carbs. I denied myself crucial fat, which is what my brain needed for fuel. I'm surprised that my memory was as good as it was!

Here is a quick breakdown of my T.A.S.K. method to a healthy, abundant diet, or what I call the Abundant Diet 365 (translation: how you should eat all year long). I love acronyms, as they are simple to teach and easy to remember. I even named my clinic Simply Health Institute because if it's not simple, people won't do it! The *T* is for "task," *A* is for "add," *S* is for "subtract," and *K* is for "keep." Let me walk you through what this looks like.

Task

I give patients the task of tracking the following nine things to bring awareness to what is missing in their diets:

1. **Macros**: These are proteins, carbs, and fats. There are two free apps that allow you to track macros effortlessly: www.myfitnesspal. com and www.cronometer.com. All you have to do is input into the app what you eat.

   a. Proteins: Most people need to be eating 1 gram of protein per pound of ideal body weight, per day. If you're at your ideal weight of 125 pounds at 5 feet 5 inches, and want to maintain weight and not lose muscle mass, then you should be eating

125 grams of protein per day. Let me give you an example of what this looks like: Four ounces of meat is 30 grams of protein, as is six ounces of fish. Four ounces of meat is approximately the size of your palm. If that 125-pound woman needs to eat 125 grams of protein per day, divided over three meals, then she should eat approximately 42 grams of protein per meal. That's a fist and a half of meat, or 6 ounces per meal. Sounds simple, huh? Unfortunately, this is the number one thing that both men and women are deficient in, unless they are tracking their protein.

b. Carbs: You need to track how many net grams of carbohydrates you are eating a day. Net grams are calculated by taking the total grams of carbs eaten, and subtracting out the grams of fiber. Ninety-two percent of the population is metabolically unhealthy. Most people should be eating less than 100 grams of carbs a day. If you're very insulin resistant, you may need to eat 50 to 75 grams instead, but everyone is different! If you don't need to lose weight, and you have no issues with blood sugar or insulin, then you're probably okay to continue eating the number of grams you are currently at. Unfortunately, most people eat carbohydrates too high in proportion to their metabolic needs, throwing themselves into insulin resistance.

c. Fats: The grams of fats ingested per day will vary. This is one that takes a little more time to calculate and is a little more nuanced. I will say that you should be getting a serving of fat at EVERY meal: that is a tablespoon of olive oil or up to half of an avocado. The APOA2 gene governs how fast you burn saturated fat. It also explains why some people do not lose weight on a ketogenic diet. As it turns out, I have a single mutation of this gene and do not need as much saturated fat as someone who does not have a gene mutation.

2. **Colors of the rainbow**: The second parameter to track is the colors of the rainbow in regard to the plant-based foods you are eating on a daily basis. You need to be eating one serving of fruits or vegetables in each color category; for example, one red food, one orange, one yellow, one green, one purple, and one tan. I will include lists of examples of fruits and vegetables in each color category in the resource page for this book, which can be found at www.energizedthebook.com/resources. The goal is to bring awareness to

see if there is one color of fruit or vegetable you are simply not getting on a daily basis. That's where you start—by adding that color of fruit or vegetable to your diet each day.

3. **Servings of fruits and vegetables**: The third parameter to track is the number of servings of fruits and vegetables you are eating on a daily basis. You should be eating eight to ten servings of fruits and vegetables per day, with a higher proportion of those servings being vegetables. One serving is one cup of leafy green vegetables, or half of a cup of solid vegetables. If you were to eat one apple, one orange, and one banana, that would equal six servings for the day. If you are hitting ten servings, you will likely be ingesting the optimal amount of fiber per day, which is at least 25 grams for women and 38 grams for men. There are two types of fiber: soluble and insoluble. Soluble fiber dissolves into a gel-like substance that is important to help capture and remove toxins and cholesterol from the body. Insoluble fiber is not digested by the body, nor absorbed into the bloodstream. Instead, it forms the bulk of stools in the body, acting as a broom, sweeping waste along and aiding evacuation. Foods highest in soluble fiber include black beans, lima beans, brussels sprouts, avocados, sweet potatoes,

and broccoli. Foods highest in insoluble fiber include oat bran, beans, lentils, legumes, berries, whole grains (especially quinoa), turnips, green peas, and okra. Some foods contain both soluble and insoluble fiber.

4. **Rotation of your foods every twenty-four hours**: The next parameter to track is if you are rotating the foods that you eat every twenty-four hours. If you're like most people, you're probably eating the same breakfast, the same lunch, and the same dinner every day. We are creatures of habit. If you don't rotate your food, you can unintentionally induce food sensitivities. Our food is fuel for our microbiome, and our microbiome is directly responsible for our immune health, as well as our mental health. When you're not fueling your microbiome with a variety of foods, you are reducing fuel for your body in the form of short-chain fatty acids. Food, particularly resistant starches, is fuel for our microbiome, and the breakdown of this food is fuel for humans in the form of short-chain fatty acids (SCFAs). In an effort to use an easier to understand descriptive term, I have nick-named SCFAs "bacterial poop." Low SCFAs not only make it difficult to lose weight, but since they are necessary to fuel our immune system, they may unintentionally increase your

risk of inducing food sensitivities. We are able to measure SCFAs using a specialty stool test that we perform in functional medicine!

5. **Pre- and probiotic foods**: Do you eat one prebiotic and one probiotic food serving every day? Resistant starches are broken down into SCFAs. These foods are also known as prebiotic foods. Here are some examples of prebiotic foods: asparagus, green banana, eggplant, garlic, Jerusalem artichoke hearts, jicama, leeks, legumes, onions, radicchio, whole grains, and dandelion greens. You also should be eating one serving of probiotic foods per day, which will provide you with good bacteria. You only need a forkful per day, but more is better in this case. Here are examples of probiotic foods: fermented vegetables like sauerkraut and kimchi, kombucha, miso, natto, pickled vegetables (like pickles), and tempeh.

6. **Number of foods eaten in one week**: How many different foods do you eat in a week? An initial goal should be at least *thirty-five different foods* every week. If you're like most Americans, you're probably eating the same ten to fifteen foods week in and week out. Consider adding two to three new foods every week until you can achieve around

thirty-five different foods. One simple way to increase the number is by varying what fresh herbs you put into a salad, such as adding dill, basil, or cilantro, or using mixed greens, which can usually get you an additional three or four foods. If you are mindful when you meal plan and grocery shop, it can be easy to achieve thirty-five different foods.

7. **Balanced plate**: The next parameter to track is whether or not you are eating a balanced plate. I have a visual of this in my mind at all times when I eat. The left half of the plate should be vegetables. The top quarter of that plate should be protein in the number of grams that you need to be eating per meal. The bottom quarter of the plate is what I call TBD, which is "to be determined," based on your needs. If you are not trying to lose weight, that bottom quarter could be grains or complex carbohydrates, like quinoa or sweet potatoes. If you're trying to lose weight, I'd encourage you to make that bottom quarter of the plate additional vegetables or low sugar fruits, like berries or melon. Then off to the side of the plate, you should have a good serving of fat, like a tablespoon of olive oil, or up to half of an avocado. Lastly, you need a serving of Omega-6 fatty acids every day in a 4:1 ratio to the Omega-3 fatty acids

you eat. Best sources of Omega-6 foods that are naturally in this 4:1 ratio are walnuts and flax seeds. Other good choices of Omega-6 foods are safflower oil or tofu, but be sure to eat organic and nongenetically modified soy.

8. **Know your pH level**: The next thing to track is pH. This is done simply by using salivary or urine pH strips. Your pH should optimally be 7.4 or greater. You need to be eating more of a plant-based diet to be alkaline, whereas an acidic state will be inflammatory and catabolic, meaning you will be breaking down muscle, which you don't want! Highly acidic foods that can result in inflammation include: alcohol, sugar, coffee, tea, chocolate, wheat and grains, beef, chicken, and pork. Foods that are considered alkaline that help reduce inflammation include: fruits like apricots, apples, bananas and avocados; vegetables like asparagus, broccoli, and carrots; gluten-free grains like brown rice and quinoa; almonds; and leafy greens like lettuce, spinach, and kale.

9. **Eating windows, aka intermittent fasting**: All adults and most children should be eating two to three meals in a twelve-hour window. Some people, like those with dementia or blood sugar imbalances, will need to eat in shorter windows; for example,

two meals every six to eight hours. The exception is newborns and infants.

Let's review the nine things I would like you to track:

1. Macros
2. Colors of the rainbow
3. Servings of fruits and vegetables
4. Rotation of your foods every twenty-four hours
5. Pre- and probiotic foods
6. Number of different foods eaten in one week
7. Balanced plate
8. pH
9. Eating windows

Add

Now that you've tracked, the next step is to add in things that you are missing. Pick your top three things to focus on over the next several weeks, and add them in one at a time. Simple, huh?

Subtract

After you have successfully tracked your food and then added back in what you were missing, so that you're nourishing your body, the next step is to subtract. This is also known as an elimination diet. There are so many of these on the market, and they all work essentially the same: by identifying what foods are inflammatory for you. The goal is to remove the most common inflammatory foods for a period of twenty-one days. This does take some preparation. I always tell my patients to pick a time frame in which they are not traveling and don't have a special event, like a birthday or wedding, so that they will have more time to meal prep and won't be tempted.

For the faint of heart, I recommend a two-food elimination diet, which consists of removing gluten and dairy, as these are the top two inflammatory foods. If you have autoimmune disease, you should *not* be eating gluten or dairy, ever—period, end of story. For those who are up for more of a challenge, I recommend a four-food elimination diet, which includes removing gluten, dairy, sugar, and soy. These are the next most inflammatory foods.

But, really, I think most people should be able to eliminate the top-ten troublesome foods for twenty-one days, which are:

- alcohol
- artificial sweeteners
- caffeine
- corn
- dairy
- eggs
- peanuts
- soy
- sugar
- gluten

Sound simple? Take these foods out for twenty-one days, and don't cheat. It's only twenty-one days! If you focus on succeeding, you will! If you focus on messing up, or think that you can't do it, guess what? You will fail.

Those who have arthritis should consider removing nightshades, which include tomatoes, peppers, potatoes, and eggplant. Take them out to see if your arthritis improves. I seem to have a sensitivity to both peppers and tomatoes, and don't eat them in their raw form very often, as eating them can trigger a flare-up of my arthritis.

Others will have sensitivities to lectins. Lectins are found in high levels in beans, peanuts, lentils, tomatoes, potatoes, eggplant, wheat, and other grains. Dr. Steven Gundry has written extensively about this. If you're interested in seeing if lectins are a trigger for you, you can consider doing a trial elimination of these foods for twenty-one days.

Two other special considerations are histamines and oxalates. You can drive yourself crazy by removing too many foods. So first do a ten-food elimination diet. Most of my patients will lose eight to ten pounds just by doing an elimination diet. Don't worry if you don't have weight to lose! You won't lose weight as the diet does not restrict calories. If you don't see any improvement with a ten-food elimination diet alone, then consider first removing high-histamine foods followed by high-oxalate foods. High-histamine foods include alcohol and fermented beverages, fermented foods, and dairy products, such as yogurt and sauerkraut, dried fruits, avocados, eggplant, spinach, processed or smoked meats, fish, and shellfish. High oxalate foods include green, leafy vegetables, especially spinach, soy, almonds, potatoes, beets, tea, rhubarb, and cereal grains.

Remember that the goal is to eat abundant and diverse whole foods. The Abundant Diet 365 ensures you're eating at least thirty-five or more foods per week, so you don't limit the number of short-chain fatty acids that your body makes, as this can be detrimental to your immune and mental health.

A word on testing for food sensitivities: I strongly recommend this for two populations—children and those who have an autoimmune disease. Here is why: with children, who oftentimes have a limited diet, you do not want to limit their diets any further. With autoimmune disease, you may not always see an increase in symptoms when reintroducing foods if the autoimmune disease is one that doesn't manifest in symptoms—for example, Wegner's granulomatosis, which causes kidney dysfunction.

I once tested a child who had autism and ADHD. He tested as having a severe sensitivity to oranges, which he ate a lot of. Four weeks later, after removing oranges, he came in for a follow-up. His hyperactivity was gone, he made eye contact, and he was able to converse for several sentences! He had done neither of these things prior to removing the oranges. It can be that profound! Testing, however, does come with both false positives and negatives, while removing foods and then reintroducing them is 100 percent accurate.

Keep

This leads us to the final letter in T.A.S.K.—*K*, or "keep." On day twenty-two, you will add back in the food that you miss the most. You should eat that food three times on day twenty-two, but then stop for the next three full days. During those three days, you are to watch for a recurrence of any of the symptoms you were having—joint pain, fatigue, skin breakouts, or significant weight gain. If you do not react to that food, you may continue to eat it. If you do react to that food, then remove it for an additional month or two. After you add in one food, you add in the next food, then the next, and so on. It will take you about a month to add all these foods back in if you do the 10-food elimination diet.

If I had to pick one diet that's close to one-size-fits-all, I would say it's the Mediterranean diet, as long as you ensure you're eating an adequate amount of protein. Unfortunately, the keto diet is probably only appropriate for approximately 20 percent of the population. It is a must for those with any form of cognitive decline or seizures, as fat fuels the brain and makes your mind sharper. Believe it or not, eating keto can make you gain weight! You just have to eat enough fat to do so. Keto should be considered for certain forms of cancer, such as glioblastoma. A study showed that combining keto and radiation was superior to radiation alone in those with glioblastoma.

For those of you who want to lose weight and/or have suboptimal blood sugar levels, I strongly encourage the use of a continuous glucose monitor (CGM) for at least two weeks. They are available through pharmacies with a prescription. Cost is approximately $70 for one sensor if you use the GoodRx app. They are easy to insert, and give you continuous glucose readings throughout the day. Optimal glucose levels are as follows:

- fasting blood sugar should be below 86
- 1 hour after a meal should be under 140
- 2 hours after a meal should be below 120
- 3 hours after a meal should be back to baseline, or less than 86

Many of my patients have found CGMs extremely valuable, allowing them to determine what is contributing to blood sugar elevations throughout the day. The most common things people report causing these blood sugar elevations are:

1. Eating too many carbs, especially those that are not balanced with proteins and fats. Add a little good fat to that oatmeal you eat in the morning so you don't see your blood sugar rise.

2. Being stressed will increase cortisol, which will also increase your blood sugar.

3. Eating foods that are inflammatory for you. For example, you could be eating a perfectly

healthy food, like quinoa, but it may be inflammatory to you. If quinoa is escalating your blood sugar, and sweet potatoes are not, then you want to forego eating quinoa for twenty-one days and reassess.

If you wanted to experiment with keto, I recommend you purchase a Keto-Mojo meter, which measures both blood sugar and ketones. To be "in keto," you want to have your ketones at least above 0.5, which is considered mild ketosis, but preferably you should fall between 1.5 and 2.9. Being in ketosis too long will ultimately decrease your ability to detoxify, which is why I have my patients cycle out of ketosis periodically.

Case Study

The best example of having someone eliminate symptoms almost entirely with an elimination diet was a thirty-eight-year-old professional woman with rheumatoid arthritis who ate a typical, standard American diet. After six weeks on an elimination diet, she lost thirty pounds, and all her symptoms went away; her skin cleared, her joint pain resolved, and she stopped needing a stimulant in the morning for her sleep disorder. She'd been diagnosed with benign hypersomnia, but it made me wonder if this was even the correct diagnosis. Perhaps diet should have been tried first? Now, I'm not saying that all sleep disorders will improve with diet alone, but it certainly can't hurt, and in her instance, she was able to stop using stimulants.

I can't tell you how many people have come to me who have been prescribed Ozempic or another GLP-1 agonist for weight loss, but have not been informed on proper nutrition. The data is clear: 66 percent of people who stopped GLP-1 agonists will regain the weight they lost. The odds are not in your favor, especially if you are not eating healthily. The healthier you eat, the less junk food you will crave.

When my liver started to fail, we were living abroad in the Middle East in Qatar. The initial symptoms were severe right upper-quadrant pain. This pain seemed to subside a bit, but then the profound fatigue I had intermittently experienced the prior two decades resurfaced, along with muscle weakness after exercise.

I learned that my liver enzymes were five times the normal level. I knew something was wrong. The doctors in Qatar were recommending a liver biopsy, but I knew they would do it without an anesthetic, and there was no way I was having a biopsy without any form of anesthetic! Subsequently, I decided to get a second opinion from gastroenterologists at Massachusetts General Hospital. These doctors strongly felt I had autoimmune hepatitis. Autoimmune hepatitis carries a 50 percent mortality in three to five years if one does not take steroids.

We were due to move back to the United States for me to start my first functional medicine job. Back then, I had a little bit of knowledge about functional medicine, but not enough to treat myself.

Prior to the move, we took a celebratory trip to Sri Lanka, renting a villa with a pool across the street from the beach. We spent our mornings drinking coffee on the veranda, eating a long, leisurely breakfast, followed by a morning swim in the pool, lunch on the beach, and then swimming in the ocean.

I will never forget the squeals of my children as they did cannonball after cannonball into the pool, saying, "Watch me, Mama! Watch me!" I should have been laughing and having the time of my life. I should have felt excited for our future, and proud of how far we'd come. In those beautiful, picturesque moments, I should have felt so alive. But all I felt was dread, and all I could think about was after the long struggle to have these amazing children, I was going to leave them without a mommy. I was worried that my children would not have a mommy to see them graduate high school or college, see them get married, or see them have their own children. Children I would never get to sing the lullaby "Hush Little Baby" to, as I had done for their parents.

After this trip, I made the conscious decision not to let my children grow up without a mommy!

I undertook a functional medicine approach with the help of a functional medicine doctor with whom I'd started to train earlier in the year. He guided me through a very simple diet/lifestyle protocol. By removing gluten and dairy, my liver function normalized, and my rapidly rising antinuclear antibody nearly normalized. Ten years have passed, and I have never been diagnosed with autoimmune hepatitis, nor have I ever been on steroids. In those ten years, I have helped over 10,000 patients reverse their symptoms. With this book I hope to prevent needless suffering in millions!

Diet + Nutrients!

The first *D* includes nutrients. A word about nutrients, or vitamins and minerals: Back in 1936, the US Senate warned the American public that they should supplement with a multivitamin because our soil was depleted. I can only imagine this soil depletion has worsened over the past eight-plus decades.

Case Study

Before I dive into vital nutrients that are often depleted in most adults, I want to share a case with you to highlight the impact vitamin and mineral deficiencies can have on your health.

I had a fifty-four-year-old woman come in complaining of fatigue and muscle weakness. By the time she came to see me, she had already seen several specialists. First, she went to her family doctor with these complaints. When her family doctor found her to have muscle weakness, she sent her to a neurologist.

The neurologist was concerned she had MS—or worse, ALS! He ordered an MRI and then an EMG, which is a nerve conduction test. All he could tell her was that she had confirmed weakness on EMG, but he had no idea why. Can you imagine going from healthy to suddenly developing fatigue and muscle weakness, to being told nothing's physically wrong?

When she came to see me, I took her through my 3-D protocol, which includes doing an in-depth intake. The intake involves asking about things that most doctors don't bother to consider, such as birth history and social history, and even adverse childhood events, which can affect our ability to regulate cortisol. After this detailed intake, I did a thorough exam, confirming she was indeed weak.

I ordered labs, including a full nutrient panel, and started supplements to support some of the key nutrients that I suspected were deficient. These nutrients were the vitamins and minerals that fuel our mitochondria. I also taught her my T.A.S.K. method to the Abundant Diet 365.

Unsurprisingly, her labs showed deficiencies in carnitine, CoQ10, and B12. These are all crucial vitamins that are needed to make our energy, or ATP (adenosine triphosphate). Typically, they are deficient in vegetarians that are not being mindful of nutrient intake or supplementing. However, this patient was not a vegetarian, meaning I needed to explore the other Ds to determine why she had these deficiencies. Within three months, she had recovered 80 percent of her fatigue and muscle weakness, and by six months, she had fully recovered.

Once I identified these deficiencies, it was important to identify what was making her deficient. Was her intake inadequate? If not, then she needed to supplement for three full months, as well as track what she was eating. Both MyFitnessPal and Cronometer apps will track vitamins and minerals. As much as I'd like to say you could supply all your nutrients through your diet, it's simply not possible, even if you are eating a diet of all whole foods. That's why I recommend a multivitamin and mineral for each and every person, from infancy on up, with the dose that's appropriate for your age and weight. I always recommend third-party tested supplements to ensure they contain what they say they do, and to ensure they are not contaminated with heavy metals!

So if this patient was ingesting meat, which is high in all three of her deficiencies, the next step would be looking at how she was digesting and absorbing her food.

Deficiencies

When I first started in functional medicine in 2013, most patients had an average of three to five nutrient deficiencies. Now, the average adult I test has five to seven nutrient deficiencies. The younger the patient, the more deficiencies. Many twenty-year-olds are coming in with anywhere from ten to fifteen vitamin and mineral deficiencies, which can be a major trigger for many symptoms, the main one being fatigue.

What are the common nutrient deficiencies? Let's talk about those first, and then the ones that are depleted in people who experience fatigue.

The top three deficiencies include vitamin D, magnesium, and zinc. Other common nutrient deficiencies are B12, folate, B6, B2, NAD, vitamin E, iron, selenium, and vitamin C. These are what I check for when I run my nutrient panel on all the patients with whom I work. Vegetarians are prone to deficiencies in vitamin D, Omega-3 fatty acids, carnitine, B12, calcium, iron, and zinc.

The nutrients important for mitochondrial health include all the B vitamins, carnitine, CoQ10, Omega-3 fatty acids, zinc, vitamin C, and magnesium.

The less healthy you eat, the more vitamin and mineral deficient you likely will be. This leads to my theory of why so many people have low energy, or have subtly acclimated to lower levels of energy. Many of us are born with the same vitamin and mineral deficiencies our parents have. Over time, if you're not ingesting a whole-food diet AND supplementing, you become further deficient. Then sprinkle in a little stress. Stress depletes magnesium and B vitamins very quickly. Now add exposure to everyday toxins, like air pollution, chemical products you use for cleaning your house, and even common, everyday beauty products. These toxins damage our mitochondria, which are needed to make energy. And with age, our number of mitochondria decline. This further depletes our energy.

To recap: Vitamin and mineral deficiencies prevent you from making energy efficiently. Then, as stress causes you to deplete these vitamins and minerals, energy is even harder to produce. After age forty, the number of mitochondria you make goes down in number. Exposure to toxins damages your mitochondria, which are particularly prone to this damage because our mitochondrial DNA is not protected in histones as is the rest of our DNA. This makes it much more prone to toxins. By the way, all our mitochondrial DNA comes from our mothers, which is why I always say that if you're tired, blame your mother.

Ultimately, it is mitochondrial dysfunction that leads to fatigue. However, it all starts with vitamin and mineral deficiencies, high stress, and toxin exposure. This is why I address these other areas in my 3-D protocol for every patient. This is *my* theory of fatigue and how *I* approach it.

Start by eating an adequate diet and supplementing with nutrients, as necessary, based on your testing. Here are the core foundational supplements I recommend for every adult: I start with a multivitamin/mineral, vitamin D3 with K2, Omega-3 fatty acids, and a good probiotic (my current favorite is Megasporebiotic, as well as magnesium. Any additional vitamins and nutrients I recommend are dependent on your deficiencies. For more information on supplements, brands, and dosing, please refer to www.energizedthebook.com/resources, where you can download all the resources that go along with this book.

Summary

The T.A.S.K. method allows you to **determine what your body needs to eat** by having you track nine different areas. These areas include macros (or proteins), servings of fruits and vegetables, colors of the rainbow, rotation of your foods every twenty-four hours, number of foods you eat in any given week, pre- and probiotic foods being eaten, pH levels, balanced plate when eating, and eating windows, aka intermittent fasting.

The biggest diet mistakes most people tend to make are not eating a balanced plate, not prioritizing protein, and not eating a wider variety of foods, preventing their bodies from producing those crucial short-chain fatty acids.

The first two steps in rectifying these mistakes are adding in the items that you're lacking and prioritizing protein, at the very least. Once you are well under way in nourishing your body with my Abundant Diet 365, you will need to implement a twenty-one-day elimination diet, removing the most troublesome foods. Don't forget to reintroduce the foods you remove! Lastly, the core five supplements I recommend for adults are multivitamins/minerals, vitamin D3 with K2, probiotics, Omega-3 fatty acids, and magnesium.

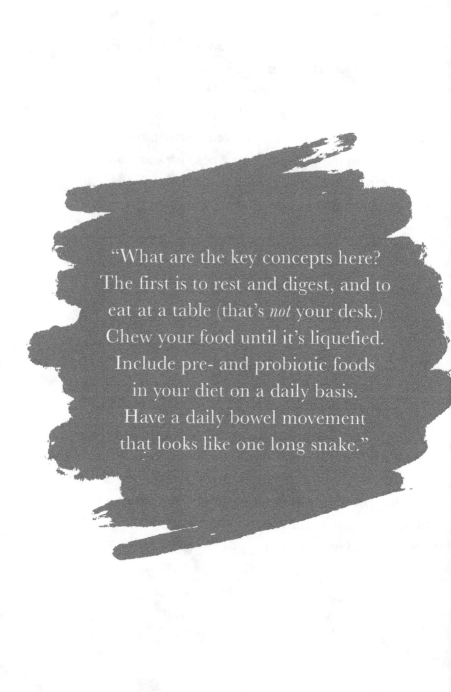

"What are the key concepts here? The first is to rest and digest, and to eat at a table (that's *not* your desk.) Chew your food until it's liquefied. Include pre- and probiotic foods in your diet on a daily basis. Have a daily bowel movement that looks like one long snake."

Chapter 2

Digestion

T he second *D* in my 3-D Energy Protocol is digestion. By this, I actually mean the microbiome, along with proper digestion.

What is the microbiome? The microbiome is all the bacteria in your large intestine; this word can also refer to bacteria found in other cavities, such as in our mouths, sinuses, and, in women, our vaginal canals. Most commonly, we are speaking about the microbiome in our large intestine. There's more DNA in our bodies from our bacteria than our own DNA! The microbiome can influence how our immune system functions through its own influence on our gut-associated lymphoid tissue (GALT). It can also influence our mental health, as nearly 70 percent of our serotonin is made by our enteric nervous system. According to the National Institutes of Health, the enteric nervous system is the largest and most complex unit of the peripheral nervous system, with approximately 600 million neurons releasing a multitude of neurotransmitters to facilitate the motor, sensory, absorptive, and secretory functions of the gastrointestinal tract.

The food that is presented to our bacteria is broken down and becomes fuel for us in the form of short-chain fatty acids. If you eat a limited number of foods per week, and don't rotate your foods, you will narrow your ability to produce short-chain fatty acids, which can affect your immune system and mental health. That's why it's important that you eat thirty-five or more different foods per week.

Case Study

Low Short-Chain Fatty Acids Result in
Psychiatric Hospital Admission

I had a really serious case that highlights the importance of our microbiome. A fifty-two-year-old woman booked an appointment with me, but before she could make it to this appointment, she was admitted to a psychiatric hospital and ended up on four different psychiatric medications. This woman had followed an elimination diet to support a family member. She felt great while on the diet, but was eating the same foods every day for *thirty days*. When she started to reintroduce foods, she developed abdominal pain, as she had inadvertently caused food sensitivities. This pain triggered her underlying anxiety, and because she wasn't producing serotonin as she used to, this further triggered her anxiety. This was the most severe case I had seen that happened as a direct result of restricting a diet to so few foods for so long.

I often reference the documentary *The Gut Movie* to my patients. The producer of this movie was an Australian who ate a standard Australian diet that was not very healthy. He had his stool tested prior to embarking on an experiment in which he flew to Namibia and lived with the indigenous people, eating only the whole foods that they ate, for one full week. At the end of the week, his stool was retested. His microbiome went from an inflammatory profile to an anti-inflammatory one in just seven days! You *can* reset your microbiome by what you eat *and* influence your health in a very short time period. That is why diet is the first step of my protocol, as it actually feeds into the second step. No pun intended.

Obviously if it were this simple, everyone would be healthy just by eating well. Before I dive into how to optimize your microbiome, let's start with digestion. We need to rest to digest. How often do you go through the drive-through and eat on the go? If you're not eating in your car, maybe you're eating at your desk. I tell my patients they should *always* be eating at a table, not at their desks.

How can you tell if you have optimal digestion? Well, the first question you want to be able to answer is "Do you poop every single day?" Healthy adults should be pooping at least once a day, if not after every meal. I often refer to the Bristol stool chart to have people identify what a healthy poop looks like. It should look like one long snake, not like hard pebbles, and not watery. Other signs that point to poor digestion are stools that float, which means you aren't getting enough fiber. Fat droplets in your stool can mean you aren't breaking down fats, and undigested food particles could mean you may not be making enough enzymes. Belching after you eat could be a sign of low OR high stomach acid. Believe it or not, in the majority of people whom I treat, belching is a sign of *low* stomach acid.

How many times do you chew each bite of food? Chewing gives our brain time to communicate down to our stomach to release hydrochloric acid so that we can break down the protein we are eating. Additionally, chewing allows for digestion to begin in the mouth through the release of salivary amylase, which breaks down carbohydrates. Ideally, you want to chew your food until it's completely liquefied.

How many of us gulp down our meals to race off to the next thing? A fun experiment I conduct is asking people to take one square of high quality organic dark chocolate and allow it to dissolve in their mouths without chewing. Can you allow it to dissolve without chewing? Really savor it? It's harder than you think! We should be chewing each bite until its liquefied *and* thoroughly enjoying each bite of food while we're resting and digesting at a table.

All of us should undergo a 5-*R* approach to ensure good digestion, remove triggers for inflammation, and optimize our health. The five *R*s are:

- Remove
- Replace
- Repopulate
- Repair
- Rebalance

Remove

This entails removing anything that is a trigger for inflammation; namely, the inflammatory foods I wrote about in chapter 2, as well as "gut bugs" or pathogens like bacteria, yeast, and parasites. It can also include removing medications like ibuprofen and unnecessary antibiotics. According to the CDC, 28 percent of antibiotics prescribed are not necessary.

I have my patients do a functional medicine stool test to identify these pathogens so that we can target them. However, as with all my protocols, by combining their symptoms, history, and labs, I can usually reverse engineer the process and do not always order a stool test. A good gut-healing protocol is typically six to eight weeks in length. I treat the pathogens with herbals in most cases, but when it comes to yeast, I also use prescription antifungals.

Yeast, parasites, and bacteria can have proteins that resemble protein in our body and, in the right person, can trigger our immune system into falsely attacking this protein in our body. In arthritis sufferers, it can be their joints, or with people who have ulcerative colitis, it can be their colon. This is called molecular mimicry. Klebsiella pneumonia is one such bacteria that has been associated with triggering the autoimmune disease ankylosing spondylitis.

I typically also recommend using a biofilm disruptor, in addition to an antimicrobial, to support the breakdown of the biofilm that many bugs form around themselves so the antimicrobial actually works. In addition, I recommend a gentle binder because when you're killing off pathogens, they can harbor heavy metals and other toxins. When you get a big dump of toxins into your system, you can be made to feel worse. Typically, the binders are taken in between meals so you don't bind up essential nutrients, medications, or supplements.

Replace

1. Stomach Acid

How do you assess whether you're making enough stomach acid or not? That's a great question. I have my patients first do a baking-soda test. First thing in the morning, you mix one-half teaspoon of baking soda in eight ounces of water. Drink this eight-ounce glass of water slowly. When you finish, set a timer. If you burp within three minutes, this suggests that you make enough acid. On the flip side, if you don't burp within three minutes, then you may not be making enough stomach acid. I always ask that you repeat this test two to three times.

If you flunk the baking-soda test, the next step is what I call the betaine challenge, in which you buy a high-quality betaine HCL supplement. For information on where to buy, please refer to the resource guide available at www.energizedthebook.com/resources. You take one betaine HCL capsule at the start of a protein-containing meal and wait to see if you develop heartburn. If you don't get heartburn, then you're not making enough, and therefore need supplemental acid. With the next meal, you can increase the dose to two capsules. If you're still not developing heartburn, then the following day you can increase to three capsules. I recommend that most people stop at three capsules, because taking too much acid can lead to gastritis or esophageal erosions, which we do not want. If you're under the age of sixty-five, by implementing my 3-D protocol, you'll usually resume making enough acid.

2. Digestive Enzymes

If you have undigested food particles or have an auto-immune disease, you need digestive enzymes. Specialty stool tests can also assess whether one produces enough pancreatic enzymes. I like my patients' pancreatic elas-tase values to be up over 500. Otherwise, I recommend that they begin supplementation with digestive enzymes. For a list of the enzymes that I recommend, please refer to www.energizedthebook.com/resources.

3. Bile Salts

If you do not have a gallbladder OR observe oily stool or oil drops in the toilet, you need supplemental bile salts; that is, ox bile. I also use Tudca, which ensures that you can recycle and produce new bile, which is an energy-intensive process for the body. If your liver and your gallbladder are overburdened or sluggish, creating new bile becomes even more difficult. Tudca also ensures you make primary bile salts. These are preferable to secondary bile salts, which are inflammatory, particularly to the brain.

4. Immune function

This is measured by secretory IgA (SIgA). A low SIgA means that there's a low immune response in the intestines. In this instance, I may recommend a colostrum-containing product. A high SIgA means that there's immune hyper-activity. Typically, a 5-R approach will normalize the secretory IgA, regardless if it is low or high.

Repopulate

Repopulating your microbiome is accomplished by eating probiotic foods: fermented foods, like kimchi and kombucha, and supplementing with probiotics. Most probiotics will stop exerting an effect if they are stopped after seven days. Spore-based probiotics, over time, will help repopulate the portion of the microbiome that was wiped out by antibiotics!

Repair

This refers to repairing intestinal permeability, aka leaky gut. Intestinal permeability has been well studied, particularly in its relation to autoimmune disease. The theory is that there are three components to autoimmune disease: genetic predisposition, a trigger, and intestinal permeability. Heal the intestinal permeability, and you can put the autoimmune disease into remission.

The triggers can be remembered by the word "STAINS." The first *S* stands for sleep and stress, the *T* for toxins. *A* is for adverse or inflammatory foods, *I* for infection or microbiome, *N* for nutrient deficiencies or excess, and the last *S* is for being sedentary or solitary. Any of these can trigger intestinal permeability, aka leaky gut. For the record, gluten causes intestinal permeability in everyone for four to six hours after it is ingested. If you are consuming gluten all day, then you have a leaky gut *all day*! This may not be a problem if you do not have autoimmune disease or a predisposition to it, but it is a problem if you do. I advise all patients with autoimmune disease to avoid gluten for life.

The top agents I have used to repair intestinal permeability include glutamine, fish oil, and zinc carnosine. More recently, I have seen even better results with a peptide known as BPC-157. My practice has been transitioning away from chronically ill patients to those seeking longevity with a desire to live long, well.

Peptides are short chains of amino acids—less than fifty amino acids, to be exact. Amino acids are breakdown products of protein. There are over 7,000 naturally occurring peptides in our bodies. The most well-known peptide is insulin. The peptides that have been all over the media are the GLP-1 agonists for weight loss (like Ozempic). Peptides are signaling molecules, and they have been found to have many benefits. Unfortunately, they decline with age.

I have had patients' autoimmune-disease flare-ups reverse in as little as a couple of months by using oral BPC-157 for at least three months. It is considered the Swiss Army knife of peptides. I hope to soon write another book on longevity, which will include a lot more on peptides. If you want to learn more about peptides, follow me on social media: Instagram @drrajka or www.facebook.com/drrajka.

Some stool tests measure zonulin, which is a marker for intestinal permeability. However, if zonulin is negative, it does not mean that intestinal permeability is not occurring, because it's just one measure in time. I assume that all people who come in with symptoms and disease have intestinal permeability.

Rebalance

This refers to quality sleep, stress modification, movement, and quality relationships. I will write more about this in the chapters on sleep and stress.

Case Studies

Rheumatoid Arthritis

To highlight the importance of the microbiome, I had a woman come to me initially to consult about an MTHFR gene mutation and a history of recurrent miscarriages. She wanted to prevent further miscarriages. While she waited to see me, she developed acute rheumatoid arthritis. Fortunately, she had started an autoimmune paleo diet and was well on her way to supporting the first *D* of my 3-D protocol. Besides an autoimmune paleo diet, I had her start taking immune-boosting supplements, including vitamin D, fish oil, zinc, and probiotics. Then I ordered a stool test, which revealed Klebsiella pneumonia. Both Crohn's disease and ankylosing spondylitis are triggered by Klebsiella pneumonia. If you treat the bacteria, you can oftentimes put the autoimmune disease in remission, which was the case with this young lady.

I hadn't seen her for eighteen months. When she resurfaced, I was initially worried that she'd had no improvement, which would explain why she hadn't followed up. When I asked her about her arthritis, she said, "I feel like I never had rheumatoid arthritis!" It had gone into remission after she followed my 3-D protocol. She was now seeing me to go through her extensive genetics, which were very revealing, and which I'll disclose in my next chapter when I review my last *D*: detox.

This is yet another example of how significant a role the microbiome can play in a disease process.

I had another woman who, among her symptoms, was not only fatigued, but had significant bloating. She ended up implementing prebiotic foods into her diet every single day, and was amazed when just this single thing resulted in complete resolution of her bloating.

It doesn't *have* to take multiple steps or extensive testing. For some people, it's just doing the basics that will result in relief and restoration of balance.

Summary

What are the key concepts here? The first is to rest and digest, and to eat at a table (that's *not* your desk.) Chew your food until it's liquefied. Include pre- and probiotic foods in your diet on a daily basis. Have a daily bowel movement that looks like one long snake.

If optimizing the diet and focusing on some of these things I talked about—such as adding prebiotic foods, betaine, or digestive enzymes—is not enough to resolve your symptoms, then do a specialty stool test.

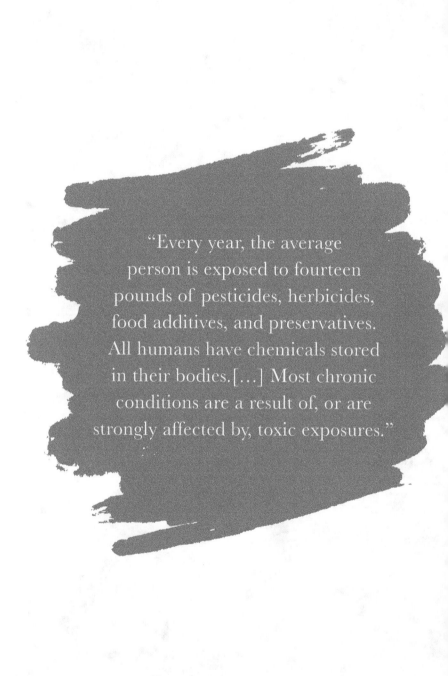

"Every year, the average person is exposed to fourteen pounds of pesticides, herbicides, food additives, and preservatives. All humans have chemicals stored in their bodies.[…] Most chronic conditions are a result of, or are strongly affected by, toxic exposures."

Chapter 3

Detox: A Dirty Little Word

W hen I talk about detoxification, I'm not talking about *woo-woo* or a quick fad. I'm talking about the natural biochemical processes that occur in our body to remove the toxins to which we are exposed. These toxins range from air pollution, to chemicals that we encounter in cleaning and personal-care products, the water we drink, and, unfortunately, the food we eat.

At every step of the way, my fatigue would start to get better, and then it would get worse. When I was forty-four, I was traveling back to the United States after my first-ever functional medicine conference. I dreaded the return trip home because it took me increasingly longer and longer to recover from the jet lag. The time it took me to recover had gone from one week, to two weeks, to three weeks, and then four! Can you imagine feeling awful and nearly nonfunctional for a full month just because you wanted to travel? This *always* happened when I would fly east on long-haul flights.

At the time, my family and I were living in Qatar. It was a lifelong dream to travel, and my husband and I longed to share the expatriate experience as a couple. We ended up in Qatar for four years longer than we had anticipated, in part due to my ongoing struggles with fatigue. Thankfully, it was a very fruitful experience, and we have many memories and good friends living across the world to show for it.

I had found the field of functional medicine and was delighted to be attending my first-ever functional medicine conference in Los Angeles. Now, that's a long-haul flight, to say the least, from Qatar to Los Angeles! I was relatively okay on arrival, and recovered my energy fairly quickly. Towards the end of the conference, I was strolling through the exhibition hall and happened upon a booth in which they were selling glutathione. The nutraceutical rep asked if I was excited to return to my children after this weeklong conference. I told him I was excited and didn't like to leave them, especially when it took me so long to recover from the jet lag.

He then told me he had a solution and handed me some of his company's samples. "Take this glutathione twice daily on an empty stomach, and start melatonin nightly."

When I returned to Qatar, it took precisely three days for me to recover from jet lag. Three days! I was absolutely astounded at going from four weeks down to three days! It seemed too good to be true. That's how important and powerful detoxification is. I continued to take the glutathione for the next six months, but then, for whatever reason, I stopped. Perhaps it was because I did not know my own genetic mutations or the ramifications of stopping...

Every year, the average person is exposed to fourteen pounds of pesticides, herbicides, food additives, and preservatives. All humans have chemicals stored in their bodies. Unfortunately, many of these chemicals have been shown to cause up to 95 percent of all cancers. Dioxins and PCBs are among the most potent causes of cancers known to man. Are you at risk? Let's talk about where these chemical toxins come from.

Dioxins and PCBs outgas from carbonless copy paper, plastics, inks, paints, furnishings, and construction glue. Xylene outgases from plastics, carpeting, furnishings, construction materials, industrial traffic exhaust, and more. Styrene outgases from our computers and many everyday plastics that hold our juices, water, soda, ketchup, peanut butter, milk, and even baby formula.

But it's not just about one exposure; it's about the total body burden. So once we're exposed, what happens to these toxins? Well, there are only two options: either they get broken down and excreted out of the body, or they're stored in our fat, bones, brain, and liver. Whether they are excreted versus stored depends on your ability to detoxify genetically, your availability of nutrients and amino acids to do so, as well as the amount of toxins you're exposed to.

Individual detoxification capability determines how much of each chemical is eliminated and how much is stored. If we use up too many detox nutrients without replenishing them, we leave ourselves vulnerable to the next environmental chemical that comes along. What are some of the effects of these toxins? Top of the list is fatigue, in addition to weight gain, diabetes, cancer, headaches, thyroid disorder, and heart disease. For the latter, think mercury. Most chronic conditions are a result of, or are strongly affected by, toxic exposures.

Where do these come from? These toxic exposures come from the air we breathe, the water we drink, the food we consume, and the products we're exposed to every day. What's the best way to eliminate toxins? Avoid them in the first place! Actually, it's to poop, pee, or sweat them out. It takes an average of twenty-six seconds for the chemicals in typical housecleaning products to enter the bloodstream. If after cleaning you can smell that clean-house smell, those cleaning products are producing chemicals that are now entering into your bloodstream.

According to studies of human exposure to air pollutants, indoor levels of pollutants may be two to five times—and occasionally more than one hundred times!—higher than outdoor pollutant levels.

Clean Water

Now let's look at sources and how to avoid them. You need to drink clean water. Unfortunately, much of our city water is contaminated. You can use EWG's tap-water source to determine how badly the water in your area is contaminated. Simply go to www.ewg.org/tapwater. The tap water in the town we live in has eight contaminants detected above health-guideline levels, including a gasoline by-product, MTBE, which occurs when gasoline tanks underneath gas stations leak into the soil.

In addition, the chlorine that is used to disinfect our water to keep us safe breaks down into a by-product called chlorine-disinfected by-products (DBPs) that are 1,000 times more toxic than chlorine. The DBPs, when heated—for example, in our showers and baths—not only absorb through the skin, but are inhaled. DPB can double the risk of rectal and bladder cancers in certain individuals. In fact, showering is infinitely more toxic to you than drinking one gallon of tap water. If you can afford one thing: buy a shower filter to filter out chlorine.

You want to also filter your drinking water. There are a variety of filters available, from simple pitchers to under-the-sink filters, to whole-house filters, such as the reverse osmosis ones. For a full list of water filters, go to www.

energizedthebook.com/resources. I often recommend the products from Clearly Filtered, www.clearlyfiltered.com.

Clean Air

We've established that our indoor air can be more polluted than our outdoor air. Then, just recently, due to uncontrolled wildfires in Canada, there are parts of the United States that have had such poor air quality you could see it color the sky! If you want to know if the air quality remains safe in your area, you can use this website to check on a daily basis: www.airnow.gov. So how *do* we get clean air, especially since our indoor air may be significantly more toxic than the outdoor air? Use an air filter. You can use an individual room filter that you move from room to room. I would recommend at least having an air filter for your bedroom where you spend many hours of the day. The top two brands I recommend are Austin Air and IQ Air. You can find links in the resource page that accompanies this book at www.energizedthe-book.com/resources.

Clean Food

What about our food? I used to say you only need to buy the foods that have been listed as the Dirty Dozen in its organic form (www.ewg.org), which would spare the expense of having to buy only all-organic produce. Meaning you could buy the Clean Fifteen foods inorganically to lower your grocery bill. However, based on current studies, one pesticide was not measured when compiling this list. That pesticide is Roundup (aka glyphosate), which is in all conventional produce. Even all California wines are contaminated with glyphosate. I recommend drinking imported wines, particularly from countries that ban glyphosate.

Clean Personal-Care Products

The horrible truth about skin care is that the average woman is exposed to up to 126 different chemical ingredients daily through skin-care products. These are readily absorbed, as our skin is the body's largest organ. According to several studies, parabens, which are synthetic preservatives found in most skin-care products, may exert serious health effects, including hormone disruption, organ system toxicity, reproductive toxicity, infertility, and birth or developmental delays.

The three chemicals you should avoid in your skin-care products, at a bare minimum, are BPA, phalates, and parabens. These chemicals can act as xenoestrogens, meaning they mimic estrogen in the body and can create a state called estrogen dominance, which we will review in the next chapter.

What is one to do? First, do an assessment of what you are actually using. There are two apps I recommend: www.thinkdirtyapp.com and EWG's skin-deep cosmetics database: www.ewg.org/skindeep. Links for both of these are also found in the online resource for this book: www. energizedthebook.com/resource.

Sadly, throughout all my twenties, I used three products that were highly toxic. The first was Dove Beauty Cream shower soap. The second was NIVEA Creme, which was even more toxic than the Dove. The third was L'Oréal makeup remover. It may have been okay had I used them only once or twice, or even for only a year. However, I utilized these products for over two *decades* before I learned how toxic they were.

Safe Cleaning Products

What about cleaning products? For the home, probably the safest thing to use is water and vinegar. Let's highlight some of the chemical toxins found in cleaning products: chlorine bleach, petroleum distillates, phenol and cresyl (found in disinfectants), nitrobenzene (found in furniture and floor polishes), formaldehyde (used as a preservative in many household products), naphthalene and paradichlorbenzene (found in mothballs), and hydrochloric acid or sodium acid sulfate (found in toilet bowl cleaners).

What is one to do? As recommended for the prior steps, do an assessment of the cleaning products that you are utilizing so that you may replace any toxic ones with safer ones. EWG has a guide to healthy cleaning, which can be found here: www.ewg.org/guides/cleaners.

Our body's main detoxification organ is our liver. All toxins that come in must undergo phase one detoxification, in which that toxin is actually broken down into an even more toxic metabolite. This process requires B vitamins such as folate, fat soluble vitamins such as vitamins A and D, antioxidants such as vitamins C and E, milk thistle, and glutathione. Once this toxic metabolite is made, it needs to be transformed into a water-loving hydrophilic molecule so we can pee, poop, or sweat it out.

This second step, called phase two detoxification, requires amino acids. Amino acids are breakdown products of protein. If not transitioning from phase one to phase two, these toxins will be trapped in a more toxic state within our bodies. That's why juice cleanses are not an ideal detox, particularly for someone who is full of toxins, because the toxins will be broken down from their original state into a more toxic metabolite. But if you are not ingesting adequate protein (which you don't while on a juice cleanse), you will not be able to convert this toxic metabolite into a water-loving molecule so that it can be excreted out of the body. The accumulation of these toxic metabolites wreaks havoc on our bodies and makes us sick. Please reconsider that juice cleanse, especially if you have never done one.

Recent studies have even shown that persistent organic chlorine pollutants are associated with an increased risk of type two diabetes. If you took a similar age and weight population of people, those with higher persistent organic pollutants had a higher risk of type two diabetes, independent of what they ate. A study published in *JAMA* showed an association between urinary BPA and obesity in both children and adolescents.

Case Study

Remember that woman who came in with rheumatoid arthritis? Why did she get better? I took her through my 3-D protocol. I advised her to eat an all-organic diet and supplied her with deficient nutrients. Then I optimized her microbiome so she could better absorb nutrients. I removed the bacteria (Klebsiella pneumoniae, in her case) that was serving as a trigger. I then had her undergo a twenty-one-day detox, which is a specific way of eating, supported with detox nutrients. The reason why this was relevant for her was that she had a double genetic mutation in the PON1 gene. This gene supports the detoxification of pesticides. By eating organic, she naturally reduced her body burden of these pesticides. She also had a significant mutation in one of her detox pathways called SOD. SOD, or superoxide dismutase, converts the free-radical superoxide to hydrogen peroxide, H_2O_2, which then needs to be further neutralized to water, or water and oxygen. This occurs via catalase and glutathione peroxidase.

Free radicals are produced every time we make ATP or energy. A small amount is good, as it helps us fight infection. Too much is bad, as it causes destruction in our bodies—and in this person's case, joint destruction. In this patient, I recommended supplementing with SOD and catalase, which further reduced her joint pain. Toxins cause free radicals in the body. This is a problem if you can't clear them.

This is why she had complete remission of her rheumatoid arthritis. By taking her through my 3-D protocol, she was able to reverse her rheumatoid arthritis and restore her energy.

Summary

You need to filter your air, filter your water, eat organic, and only use safe cleaning and personal-care products. Additionally, you want to ensure you have an adequate number of nutrients that are required for detoxification and an adequate protein intake. Adequate protein is one gram per pound of ideal body weight of protein per day, or 30 to 40 grams of protein at every meal. You may also want to consider having toxins measured. I have been fooled many a time when someone is "eating and living clean." You would expect them to have low toxin levels, but when measured, their toxins were found to be sky-high. Testing helps to pinpoint a source, as well as provides information on which specific binders are needed to remove these toxins. I use a variety of binders, which I will share in the resource page at www.energizedthebook.com/resources.

Lastly, remember my theory on fatigue: patients are born with nutrient deficiencies. These nutrient deficiencies are worsened by eating a poor diet, along with exposure to stressors, which further deplete us of crucial vitamins. Then, through lifelong exposures to toxins, our mitochondria, which make energy, are damaged, and toxin exposures further deplete us of our nutrients. It becomes a vicious cycle. That's why it is so very important to support detox so that we have properly functioning mitochondria. The key to not only a healthy life, but to infinite energy, is eliminating mitochondrial dysfunction.

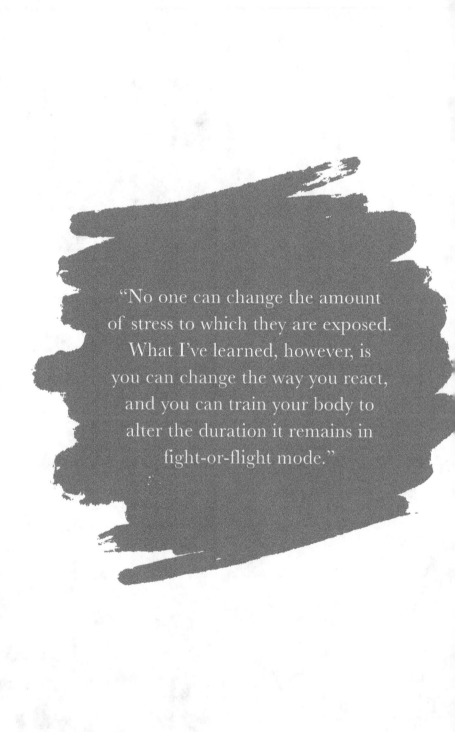

"No one can change the amount of stress to which they are exposed. What I've learned, however, is you can change the way you react, and you can train your body to alter the duration it remains in fight-or-flight mode."

Chapter 4

Stress and Hormones

W hat I told you in the beginning of my book is that I would teach you my 3-D energy protocol. What I didn't tell you is that it is actually $3D$s, $3S$s, and $3M$s or $3D+3S+3M$ = High Energy. The $3S$s are: sleep, stress, and sex (or movement!). The 3Ms are meaning in life, mindset, and time management. I will review these additional steps of the protocol in subsequent chapters, starting with stress.

No one can change the amount of stress to which they are exposed. What I've learned, however, is you can change the way you react, and you can train your body to alter the duration it remains in fight-or-flight mode. A moderate amount of stress can be beneficial, but excess stress not only results in numerous symptoms, but is also a significant factor in all chronic diseases.

In my new patient intake, I evaluate people's stress levels, the stress modification techniques they use, and the adverse childhood events they've faced. Adverse childhood events can be significant traumas a child experienced or even perceived as traumatic. In my practice I use the ACE questionnaire that consists of ten questions, each scored with a point. A higher score is correlated with a dysregulated cortisol response and an increased risk of developing chronic diseases. The influence of stress is profound.

Stressors

Sometimes, stress doesn't make its presence overtly known. Take the case of Linda, a highly successful businesswoman who approached me in her late sixties, baffled by her severe fatigue. When probed about potential stress triggers, she recounted a challenging contract she had recently finished. Although she never felt stressed, her symptoms—ranging from bloating to diarrhea, and even fatigue—spoke otherwise. This demonstrates the sometimes subtle power of stress, with symptoms not always overtly related to stress itself. Notably, there's a significant gut-brain connection which might explain why stress sometimes manifests as gastrointestinal symptoms, as it did for Linda. By following my 3-D protocol, Linda's symptoms improved rapidly, restoring her vigor.

Reflecting on Linda's case early in my functional medicine practice, I realized that while I had discussed stressors and their impact, I might not have emphasized the importance of continuous stress-resilience techniques.

As a result of this, Linda returned a few years later, grappling with fatigue that emerged after another high-stress project. She reiterated, "But, Doc, I didn't feel stressed."

Clearly, her body felt otherwise. Now, I prioritize teaching biofeedback to all our patients, a tool especially favored by executives. It offers a tangible way to discern if they've truly exited the fight-or-flight mode. Some of my patients might meditate daily for many years, but they never fully exit this fight-or-flight state, detrimentally impacting their health. Now we not only teach biofeedback, but also emphasize the necessity of consistent practice to achieve genuine resilience against stress. This should be an ongoing practice, so that when we are exposed to a stressor, we can more readily move out of fight-or-flight mode.

Cortisol

It's essential to understand the typical stress response and cortisol patterns. Cortisol should be high in the morning for alertness, and decrease gradually throughout the day, allowing us to sleep. However, consistent exposure to stressors results in sustained elevated cortisol and adrenaline levels, also thought of as our fight-or-flight response, leading to various stages of adrenal dysfunction.

The first stage of adrenal dysfunction is a result of cortisol being elevated all day long, which leaves that person feeling wired. The next stage is inversion of the cortisol curve, where cortisol is low in the morning and high at night; that leaves a person feeling tired during the day and wired at night. These people will almost always have a hard time falling asleep, and will often wake up between 2:00 and 4:00 a.m., struggling to fall back asleep. The last stage of adrenal dysfunction comes from a flattened cortisol curve, leaving that person feeling tired all day, every day. By regulating the stress response, these levels can normalize back to baseline levels.

Hormones: Adrenal, Thyroid, and Sex

The profound impact of how prior trauma can alter cortisol lifelong has been captured in the book *The Body Keeps the Score*. Stored prior trauma that alters cortisol levels can manifest as physical symptoms, particularly fatigue. Yet, when discussing stress, it's pivotal to consider all hormones—not just stress hormones. This includes the intricate relationship between thyroid hormones *and* our sex hormones—estrogen, progesterone, and testosterone.

Chronic stress can impact thyroid-hormone production, which is initiated by the release of thyroid-stimulating hormone (TSH) by the brain. TSH triggers the release of Free T4 (FT4) from the thyroid gland. For optimal release, several nutrients and conditions are required, such as selenium, zinc, iodine, low stress, and minimal toxins. In conditions of stress or toxin exposure, the inactive thyroid hormone FT4 might convert to a less useful form called Reverse T3 (RT3), instead of Free T3 (FT3), the active form, further exemplifying the body's intricate stress-adaptation mechanism.

Imagine FT4 is a paycheck: you can't do anything with a check alone until it is cashed. The cashed check should be thought of as FT3, which is the active form of thyroid hormone our body can readily use. Too much stress, and FT4 is instead converted to RT3, which is like a voided check—useless. RT3 cannot be utilized. Again, this is our body's way of preserving our metabolic function. When we're exposed to stressors, such as famine, wouldn't you want to preserve calories if you had no food? Of course, you would, and so does your body!

Along with many of my patients, I personally experienced subclinical hypothyroidism for at least a decade prior to being diagnosed. Apart from the vitamins and minerals I am most certain were depleted, it was the chronic stress and, in my case, an autoimmune component that was causing my own body to attack my thyroid. If only someone had guided me through the 3-D protocol sooner, I might not have endured such prolonged fatigue.

Now, addressing sex hormones: both men and women produce progesterone, estrogen, and testosterone. However, women produce less testosterone than men, and men produce less estrogen than women. The most frequent hormonal imbalance in women is estrogen dominance, which can result in a myriad of symptoms throughout a woman's life, such as painful periods, irregular periods, heavy bleeding, acne, tender and even fibrocystic breasts, infertility, mood swings, premenstrual depression, and hot flashes as they near menopause.

Why does estrogen dominance occur? Estrogen dominance occurs when a woman either does not clear estrogen effectively, or she is exposed to outside sources of estrogen, such as BPA, parabens and phthalates, which are all too common in women's personal and beauty-care products. Or this occurs as the production of progesterone falls during perimenopause, which makes the estrogen higher in proportion to progesterone.

Not clearing estrogen can be a result of not having adequate magnesium, antioxidants, B vitamins, or glutathione. It can also be caused by having gene mutations in those directly responsible for clearing estrogen. Some women will more readily convert some of their estrogens into either the intermediate estrogen, 16alpha-Hydroxyestrone, which is the estrogen that contributes to fibrocystic breasts and endometriosis, or more readily to 4-Hydroxyestrone or 4-Hydroxyestradiol, which can lead to DNA damage and has been associated with breast cancer. That's why it's so important to eat an abundant, nourishing diet to help with clearance and to support nutrients, which is my first D in the 3-D protocol.

Then, by supporting digestion (or the microbiome) you can further support proper estrogen clearance. There are actually bacteria that produce an enzyme called beta-glucuronidase. Beta-glucuronidase cleaves the water-loving molecule that gets attached to estrogen to allow us to poop, pee, or sweat it out when we're done utilizing it. So if this molecule is cleaved, that estrogen will enter back into circulation. This is called hepatic recirculation. It's another way that estrogen levels can be relatively high, as compared to progesterone levels. Estrogen released early in the cycle helps build the lining of our uterus. While progesterone, which is released mid-cycle onward, helps shed the lining. If we do not conceive, we have our periods. A typical, healthy estrogen-progesterone ratio is five to one (or fifty to ten). Unfortunately, I've seen extremely abnormal ratios.

Case Study

One woman whom I took care of would frequently go into manic episodes. When tested, we found that she had an estrogen of over 500, while her progesterone was down around five. That's a *big* difference, or a one hundred-to-one ratio, instead of a five-to-one ratio. Fortunately, we were able to balance her hormones, and her manic episodes subsided.

Menopause and Andropause Considerations

Men produce progesterone, but far less of it than women. Obviously, men produce more testosterone, but women produce testosterone as well. Testosterone does wane in both sexes as we age, starting around age forty. Men will often experience symptoms of andropause, and, believe it or not, these symptoms are very similar to menopausal symptoms in women! For some people, depending on how out of balance they are, this can occur much sooner. What I saw in my practice was, as women headed into perimenopause, they typically came in around their late forties. This is usually a couple of years before menopause, with the average age of menopause is fifty-one. I started to notice that this got earlier and earlier and earlier, and, soon enough, I was starting to see women in their *early thirties* with symptoms of perimenopause, and even menopause! Again, we have to consider a highly toxic environment, along with a high-stress environment, may be responsible for these symptoms being seen earlier and earlier.

The topic of hormone replacement therapy is controversial, particularly following a study, in the early 2000s, which associated certain therapies with increased cancer risk. The Women's Health Initiative study showed that a combined synthetic product—which included Premarin, a synthetic estrogen (made from horses' urine), and Provera, (medroxyprogesterone), a synthetic progesterone—was linked to a higher risk of breast and colon cancer in women. This higher risk came from a study of 10,000 women, in which eight more women out of 10,000 were identified as having these diseases. Unfortunately, what the study didn't highlight was that estrogen alone, even in synthetic form, did not cause this increased risk of breast cancer. The study did not test or utilize bioidentical hormones.

Now, I'm not here to argue the study or whether hormone replacement should have been discontinued in every single woman. But the fact remains that more women went on to develop heart attacks, memory loss, and osteoporosis because of a lack of hormone replacement after menopause. Estrogen is protective to the brain, as well as to the bones, and has even been associated with decreased risk of heart attacks. Remember, because of their higher estrogen levels, women have a lower risk of heart attack before menopause than men.

Informed Consent

In all my patients at every step of the way, optimizing diet, digestion, and detox almost always led to a better balance of hormones. If someone is truly in menopause or andropause, implementing these changes prior to hormone replacement usually results in lower levels of hormones being needed.

In my discussions with patients, we cover optimal lifestyle, stress modification, and foods, along with supplements, to support optimally balanced hormones. We may even discuss peptide support of hormone production or bioidentical hormone replacement. The choice is up to the them. While there is a risk with bioidentical hormones, it is much lower than with the use of synthetics, and when dosed correctly and monitored appropriately, they can be extremely beneficial.

Naturally, this should be monitored. Your doctor needs to be measuring your hormones regularly, starting at baseline, then six weeks later, then three months later, and then at routine intervals. Personally, I like to get blood levels to begin with, along with a urine hormone test that allows me to determine how you break down your hormones. This is important because you really need to know how hormones are broken down in order to safely replace them. For example, in a woman, if testosterone is broken down too quickly into DHT (dihydrotestosterone), it can induce male-pattern balding. Not exactly desirable for men or women! Alternatively, if testosterone is given to a man who more readily breaks this down into estrogen, it can induce "man boobs." Again, not desirable!

That said, every step in my patient's journey emphasizes optimizing diet, digestion, and detox, which often leads to hormonal balance. The choices and risks are presented to the patient transparently, ensuring they remain informed and in control.

Case Study

I recall an incident while traveling to a hormone conference in Los Angeles. I was at the car rental office for more than an hour after they had given away my car because my flight was late. While I was there, I chatted with a gentleman in his early sixties who had come back for his college reunion. He wanted to look good for this event, so he had met with a doctor who put him on testosterone. Unfortunately for this man, the testosterone led to significant weight gain around his hips and gave him "man boobs." Not exactly the effects he wanted when trying to look his best after not seeing some of his friends for so many years.

Balance

It is important to know that when you replace one hormone, it affects all the other hormones. If your adrenal gland is not functional, it will negatively affect your thyroid gland, so you must support adrenal function. This can be done with stress modification, herbals, and in some instances, it needs to be done with a low level of corticosteroids, which I rarely, if ever, have had to use.

Remember when I said that all hormones need to be monitored appropriately? That includes not only monitoring the levels and how the hormones are broken down in an individual's body, along with yearly exams by a patient's primary care physician, but also screening for typical cancers. These cancers include prostate cancer in men, breast cancer in women, and colon cancer in both men and women.

What I can tell you is that if a man or woman has their hormones in balance, there's nothing like it. I'll often hear, "I finally feel like my old self again!" Now isn't *that* the ultimate goal?

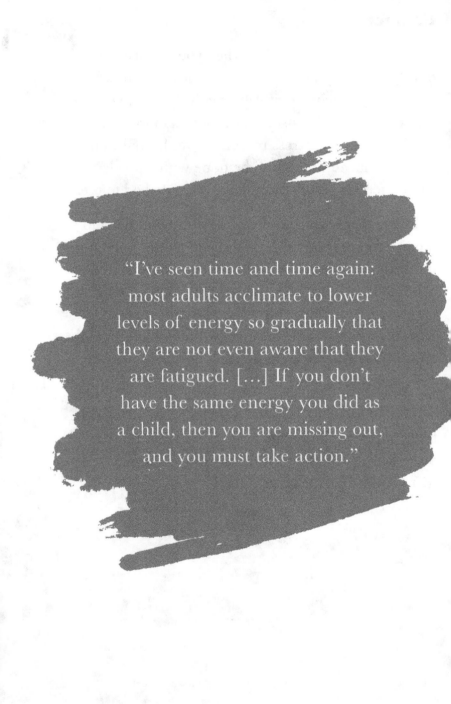

"I've seen time and time again: most adults acclimate to lower levels of energy so gradually that they are not even aware that they are fatigued. […] If you don't have the same energy you did as a child, then you are missing out, and you must take action."

Chapter 5

Sleep

If you're not sleeping, I can't help you lose weight, balance your hormones, reverse your autoimmune disease, or address any number of conditions. So let me help you sleep!

Case Study

I was seeing a teenage patient who came in with her mother, who, at only fifty-three, would forget what I said after just a few sentences. I later discovered that this memory lapse was due to her having slept only four to five hours a night for months. I remember thinking, even though she wasn't my patient, *At only fifty-three years old, she shouldn't be having these problems with her memory.* Eventually it became evident that her memory was improved, and I couldn't help but ask what had changed. She revealed she was finally sleeping eight hours throughout night.

This is the power of sleep deprivation. In a recent study of military recruits, sleep deprivation was shown to be the mental equivalent of being intoxicated. In the case of my patient's mother, it was the equivalent of her having dementia. Just imagine being able to restore your memory with adequate sleep! I have countless cases in which sleep was the main issue.

Now, you may ask, was it one trigger that led to symptoms and disease, or was it multiple? Typically, it is at least three different triggers, if not more. And the longer you've been sick? Well, you can guarantee that probably all eight triggers are causing imbalances, symptoms, and disease.

Sleep as a Concept

So before we dive into how we fix your sleep, let's talk about what *makes* you sleep. When you wake up in the morning, light striking your eyes helps reset our circadian rhythm. That's important. There are alarm clocks that will brighten your room, or people have set their shades to open with timers, but probably the best thing to do is get outside first thing in the morning. In an ideal world, you would do this at sunrise, opening your eyes to at least ten minutes of the morning light…and, no, I don't mean sunlight directly into your eyes. But don't wear sunglasses, either! Those few minutes each morning will help you reset your circadian rhythm, keep alert during the day, and fall asleep at night.

Each day, your cortisol level should rise about thirty minutes after awakening. We call that the cortisol-awakening response. Throughout the day, your cortisol should gradually go down. Imagine it rolling down a hill, with the lowest level being before you go to bed. When this does not happen, you will have disrupted sleep. When you are exposed to chronic stress, day in and day out, cortisol goes up throughout the day *and* night. This could make you feel wired and lead to difficulty falling and/or staying asleep.

Over time, chronically stressed people end up with an inversion of the cortisol curve, meaning that when they awaken their cortisol is low. This leads them to feel tired. Then, as nighttime comes about, they feel wired *and* tired. This will not only cause them to have difficulty falling asleep, but also to awaken in the middle of the night.

The levels of serotonin, melatonin, and GABA, three different chemicals in our bodies, must rise in order for us to GO to sleep. We already talked about needing morning light so that melatonin will reset. Conversely, if you're getting a lot of blue light before bed, you can completely shut down melatonin production, which makes falling asleep difficult, and quality sleep almost impossible.

GABA may not be produced adequately at night if you're deficient in magnesium and vitamin B6 because these vitamins and minerals are needed to convert glutamate into GABA. Additionally, you need serotonin, which comes from tryptophan, to rise at night. There can be any number of reasons why this conversion isn't happening, starting with insufficient protein intake (tryptophan comes from protein), insufficient ability to digest protein, or insufficient vitamins and minerals needed to convert tryptophan to serotonin, which then later gets converted to melatonin. Even genetic mutations can cause a decrease in melatonin, GABA, or serotonin.

Let Me Sleep!

Now that we've talked about what allows you to sleep, let's talk about things that can get in the way of falling asleep. If you're having difficulty falling asleep, it can be due to anxiety, not enough GABA, too much cortisol, or not enough melatonin. There are three major areas we tackle to facilitate sleep. The first is avoid blue light for at least *two hours* before bed, and if you have to be on the computer, wear complete-blue-blocking glasses. Second, you want to get your morning light in, and not only upon awakening, but throughout the day—ten minutes, several times a day—especially in regards to cortisol rising at bedtime. Finally, work on that stress response.

One of my four favorite modalities that I teach all my patients is biofeedback using HeartMath, which has been around for decades. Just by using HeartMath ten minutes before bed, you can improve the quality of your sleep by 30 percent over six to nine weeks. This is powerful! No medications needed.

You can also consider cortisol-lowering supplements. My top-two supplements to lower cortisol are phosphatidylserine and ashwagandha. Typically, you would start with 100 milligrams of phosphatidylserine about an hour before you go to bed. You can gradually increase this to 300 milligrams if one hundred is not enough. But be careful! If you take too much, it can actually be a bit stimulating. In regards to ashwagandha, usually just one to two doses will do the trick. Again, start with one, and observe what happens over the course of a week. Then you can try adding a second dose, if needed, the following week.

3:00 A.M. Awakening

What causes us to wake up at 3:00 a.m.? There are four top causes of middle-of-the-night awakening that will drive you absolutely crazy. The first cause we already alluded to, which is having an inappropriate rise in cortisol before bed, and we've already talked about how to remedy this. A surefire way to see if this is happening is to ask yourself if you have difficulty sleeping when you're away on vacation and not under the usual day-to-day stress.

The second cause is having blood-sugar dysregulation, or eating too many carbohydrates right before bed, and not combining them with proteins and fats. The simple remedy is to stop eating at least two hours before bed, and ensure that that last meal you eat, regardless of how many carbs you're eating, has protein and fat to offset those carbs. That's a simple remedy. In fact, I have some people ingest a light, high-fat snack about an hour or two before bed, and this prevents them from waking in the middle of the night.

The third cause is estrogen dominance or progesterone deficiency. I typically see this in perimenopausal women. This is the absolute worst. I can't tell you the number of women whom I put on progesterone, only to have them come in later and say they simply could not do without it to sleep! So you can increase progesterone naturally by utilizing a supplement that contains chasteberry, or you can simply add progesterone in the form of oral capsules. I prefer oral because the oral form is the one that gets converted to GABA, which is calming. Remember, we said we need GABA to increase in order to facilitate falling asleep.

The fourth and last cause of middle-of-the-night awakening is parasitic infections. If you are having GI issues, this may be something to tackle. There are plenty of herbal protocols to remedy parasites and plenty of ways to treat them with prescription medications that will allow you to get back to sleep.

For resources on anything I've mentioned, please refer to the resource guide at www.energizedthebook.com/resources.

Poor Quality of Sleep

If you're having unrefreshing sleep, it means that, no matter how you're sleeping or how much you're sleeping, you wake up unrefreshed. You want to first ensure that you don't have some sort of sleep disorder, such as sleep apnea, narcolepsy, and in some instances, benign hypersomnia. This would need evaluation by a sleep doctor to confirm the diagnosis.

But, barring any of these sleep disorders, you'll need to take a comprehensive diet/lifestyle approach and implement excellent sleep hygiene. If you are having trouble sleeping and simple measures do not facilitate sleep, you need to do everything on the following list:

1. Ensure that you have the same bedtime and wake time, whether it's during the week or weekend.

2. Get ten minutes of morning light into your eyes, preferably around sunrise, or at least right when you awaken.

3. Avoid blue lights at least two hours before bed and/or wear blue-light blockers if you must work.

4. Turn off your Wi-Fi at night! In a perfect world, you would have everything in your home hardwired.

5. Create the ideal sleeping environment. The ideal sleeping environment should be very dark, as even small amounts of light that creep out around your draperies can disrupt your sleep by a significant amount.

6. Ensure that the room temperature is cool. The best temperature for sleep is 60 to 68 degrees Fahrenheit. We sleep at 68 degrees because this is about all the cold I can tolerate. Every single one of us in our family sleeps well at night, but if it gets any hotter, nobody is sleeping well, particularly my son and my husband.

7. Avoid heavy meals before bedtime, preferably at least two hours.

8. Avoid caffeine, alcohol, or nicotine before bed.

9. Avoid stimulating activities at bedtime. You can do gentle movements, such as Tai Chi or yoga.

10. Avoid watching the news, paying bills, checking financial reports or the stock market, and arguing before going to bed. You can read entertaining material or write in a journal, as these are great activities before bed.

11. Plan at least eight to nine hours in bed because, believe it or not, you are not going to be asleep the whole time. Most people have short periods of restlessness or periods of wakefulness throughout the night.

12. Create an inviting routine before bed, one that you do in the same fashion every night.

13. Avoid getting into bed after 11:00 p.m., as sleep after midnight is not as restorative as sleep before midnight.

14. Avoid late afternoon or evening naps; naps should not be longer than forty-five minutes.

15. Do not to drink more than four to eight ounces of fluid before going to bed.

16. Don't stay in bed for more than twenty to thirty minutes after awakening.

17. Try to implement box breathing for a short period of time if you wake up before you're ready to get your day going. If you still cannot go back to sleep, then get up; you can write in a journal or sit quietly.

18. Try not to have anything plugged in at least three to six feet from the bed, as it can be disruptive to sleep. Believe it or not, there is a gene mutation which renders people more sensitive to EMFs or Wi-Fi.

19. Consider using body pillows, and be sure to use a pillow that sufficiently supports your neck.

If you're still having difficulty with unrefreshed sleep, I have my patients consider 5-HTP in the range of 50 to 150 milligrams before bedtime. This particular supplement should not be taken with common antidepressants called SSRIs. Remember, any information given in this book is for informational purposes only; it does not constitute a doctor/patient relationship.

Case Study

I had a fifty-one-year-old woman come to me; she was having unrefreshed sleep. As she was rounding out her care and transitioning to our maintenance plan, I was reviewing her supplement list to consolidate them because I only ever want people to take exactly what they need to minimize cost and make it easier to follow. When I asked if she was still taking the 5-HTP supplement that had been working quite well, she told me she'd turned off her Wi-Fi at night instead and found that to be just as effective as 5-HTP. Can you imagine a simple lifestyle measure having the same benefit as a supplement?

I can't tell you how many people come to me on addictive prescription sleep medication that has been shown to increase the risk of dementia, without ever having been counseled on simple measures, such as sleep hygiene, or offered gentle supplementation that does not carry the risk of dementia.

Case Study

I had a woman come in who was struggling with weight gain. We had taken her through many different strategies that had helped her lose weight, but she always seemed to plateau. Remember, you need to remove all triggers for inflammation, and sleep is one of them. She never reported feeling fatigued, but I had her implement exposure to sunlight three times a day for ten minutes, before 5:00 p.m., with the first time upon awakening, the second time before 12:00 noon, and the third time before 5:00 p.m. This was to help her lose weight. Mind you, she never complained of having an energy problem. She said that she felt extremely well in regards to energy, but after she had implemented the above plan for just thirty days, she said that her energy significantly improved. This correlates with what I've seen time and time again: *most adults acclimate to lower levels of energy so gradually that they are not even aware that they are fatigued.*

If you don't have the same energy you did as a child, then you are missing out, and you must take action. Low energy is one of the first signs of mitochondrial dysfunction, and this is at the crux of almost all diseases.

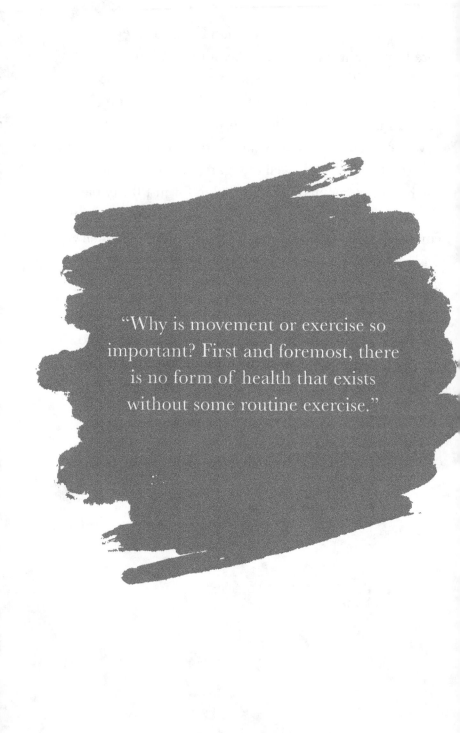

"Why is movement or exercise so important? First and foremost, there is no form of health that exists without some routine exercise."

Chapter 6

Sex! AKA Movement or Exercise

Why is movement or exercise so important? First and foremost, there is no form of health that exists without some routine exercise. After the age of forty, we lose muscle mass. If you're not doing anything to maintain it, you'll become frail, and frailty is *no bueno* when it comes to longevity.

Let's dive in to the top-three mistakes people make when it comes to exercise.

The first mistake is not exercising at all. I know this may seem puzzling to those of you who have spent hours trying to maintain or regain optimal health and energy, but I can't even tell you how many people who don't exercise have come to my office for weight loss in particular. We take them through my 3-D protocol (which is actually three *D*s plus three *S*s and three *M*s), and they never disclose that they're not exercising. It is just shocking.

So I re-review the nine-step process. And, lo and behold, they have never ever exercised.

Case Study

One high-level executive went so far as to have a gastric bypass. Can you imagine? She wasn't counseled on a proper diet, mindset, or movement prior to the surgery, or even afterwards. By utilizing my 3-D protocol, she was able to successfully take off an additional 17 pounds after she had plateaued from the gastric bypass. We re-explored what was driving this recent plateau. In her case, it was a high level of stress due to her job, as well as friction in her marriage. We met and established attainable goals to address these stressors, along with how to add in exercise despite her rigorous travel schedule for work. She is on her way now to continuing to lose weight.

The second mistake is exercising too much. Maybe you work out five days a week, or maybe you're going to CrossFit or Orangetheory, and the scale hasn't budged. You haven't noticed much difference, except maybe a little more tone, and perhaps you're getting more depleted after a year or more of doing these intense exercises so rigorously throughout the week. This level of exercise, particularly in a stressed, high-level entrepreneur or executive, further drives cortisol. Cortisol drives insulin. Insulin makes it almost impossible to lose weight. You may notice that the weight gain from high cortisol and insulin is right there in your abdomen—that tummy fat that seemingly will never go away, despite all the measures you've tried. So if you are a high-stress person, you need to go back and implement some of the strategies from the "Stress and Hormones" chapter, and then *back off on the exercise.* Take it down not one notch, but tenfold. Instead of going to Orangetheory five days a week, schedule a forty-five-minute walk, take a Tai Chi class, or do restorative yoga. You must let go of this high intensity and rigor, as it is only serving to drive up your cortisol and make it impossible to lose weight.

High cortisol is catabolic, meaning it's going to break down your muscles, which is exactly the opposite of what you're trying to achieve. I received a call from one woman who was interested in my 3-D protocol. Prior to the call, she had implemented walking instead of her CrossFit exercise, which resulted in a ten-pound weight loss in one month. It can be this significant a loss if you're inflamed and overexercising.

The third mistake people make when it comes to exercise is not having the right combination or ratio of cardio to strength training. Let's take a step back. Which form of exercise is more important for longevity? The studies are clear that strength training beats cardio, but a combination of the two packs even more of a punch.

Let's dive a little deeper into what people do wrong when it comes to cardio. The first is exercising aerobically for long periods of time. This only serves to deplete you, and is more than you need to do, especially if you're a busy executive. What's even better is HIIT (high-intensity interval training). There are studies that show as little as seven minutes a day can lead to significant health benefits, and there are several free apps that have seven-minute HIIT workouts.

When it comes to strength training, a lot of people just don't do it at all. I know I was guilty of this in my twenties and thirties, and even into my early forties. But, once I started, I got hooked! Now I've found a balance of mixing both forms of exercise.

Getting Started

How do you even start? First, figure out the least amount of time that will allow you to successfully achieve exercising at least five days a week. Maybe your schedule looks like this: Monday, Wednesday, and Friday you take a walk for fifteen to twenty minutes after meals. Walking after meals will normalize blood sugar; I've seen it happen countless times. This is one *simple* measure. You can even include your kids, your spouse, or your dog! Then, three days a week, you incorporate strength training for ten to fifteen minutes to start. There are so many different You-Tube videos you can do in regards to strength training, just by utilizing your body strength, or even adding some dumbbells that will pack a punch. I would alternate between upper-body, lower-body, and full-body workouts. If you only have time to add in strength training twice a week, do a full-body workout spaced a few days apart so you can have time to recover.

How much strength training should you do? I would start with ten minutes a day, and work your way up. Probably twenty to thirty minutes of lifting is all you need. Remember, you need time for recovery in between lifting sessions.

Here are additional tips that will make exercise a breeze:

1. Choose a form of exercise you can do anywhere. That's why walking and running for cardio is excellent, along with yoga.

2. Put it in your calendar so it is actually part of your day. Don't wait until the end of the day to incorporate it!

3. Consider investing in a low-cost app. There are so many out there. My personal favorite is the Peloton app. I use the app even more than the bicycle we purchased, although I do love the bike. If you can't afford an app, you can find plenty of workouts on YouTube that don't require any equipment. Just search for "15-minute body-weight strength training" or "15-minute HIIT workout."

4. Choose a time to work out. I suggest doing it in the morning. You'll find that it's easy to incorporate, and then it's done for the day.

5. Ensure that you stand throughout the day. Working out in the morning and then sitting

for eight hours negates the powerful effects of exercise. Sitting has become the new smoking.

6. Work out even when on the go; it is really easy to do, either at the hotel's, gym, or even in your hotel room. I always bring a fold-up yoga mat so I can exercise in the room before my meetings or conferences get started.

7. Track your progress. For three whole months, I reflected back on how much exercise I was doing. I noticed that for one full week of each of the three prior months I had not exercised at all. This correlated with times when I was out of town, which is when I started packing a yoga mat in my luggage. This ensured that I got *at least* a fifteen- to twenty-minute workout in the room. It not only made me more alert during meetings, but I felt better overall throughout the day. I continue to track my progress so that I didn't fall off the wagon.

8. Find a workout buddy. It's much more fun to work out with a friend. I can't tell you how many times I've scheduled a meet-up with a friend to walk instead of going to grab a bite to eat or a cocktail. If you don't have a friend who can walk with you, call them on the phone as you walk. You'll feel as if they're right there with you. Or listen to a great

audiobook or an inspirational YouTube talk or podcast. Preferably one about motivation!

9. Be sure you are eating an adequate amount of protein. Here are the benchmarks I ask all my patients to achieve: eat one gram of protein per pound of ideal body weight per day, divided across the meals that you eat. So a 120-pound woman would need to eat 40 grams of protein at breakfast, lunch, and dinner to maintain muscle mass. The other thing that needs to be achieved is 2.5 grams of leucine per meal after exercise. If you don't have any issues with dairy, one cup of cottage cheese gives you 2.5 grams of leucine. However, I advise people to supplement with an amino acid that contains 2.5 grams of leucine after the exercise, preferably within thirty to sixty minutes after you've worked out. For a link to my preferred forms of amino-acid complexes, please refer to www.energizedthebook.com/resources. The reason why muscle is important is because it's our currency of aging, and we need to feed our muscles to maintain them, if not to build them.

More on Peptides

Over the past year, I've been slowly incorporating peptides. They have made a huge difference in my health and well-being! As I said before, peptides are short chains of amino acids. They can be taken many different ways. There are two that I routinely use in the forty-plus crowd, especially when they want to build muscle and lean out. The first is Ipamorelin. It's a growth-hormone-releasing peptide, and it stimulates the release of growth hormones from the anterior pituitary. I combine this with CJC 1295, which is a synthetic analog of growth-hormone-releasing hormone. They both serve to increase the release of growth hormone, which then goes on to increase all the levels of our sex hormones. When used together, one fills your gas tank with fuel using growth hormones, and the other helps release them into your body.

Some of the benefits I've seen in patients with this combination of CJC and Ipamorelin are faster recovery from exercise, weight loss, improved sleep, and they more readily build muscle mass. With time, natural levels of their own sex hormones increase. For those who are on bioidentical hormones, we oftentimes have to reduce the dose when someone is on CJC/Ipamorelin. Caveat: You would never want to use this combination if someone has a known cancer diagnosis.

I typically like to dose this at 100 micrograms an hour before bed, and definitely ninety minutes after you've ingested any type of food, particularly carbohydrates. You can add a dose of 100 micrograms in the morning before eating, and then again an hour and a half after eating breakfast. As you increase the dose, for those who are stress responsive, you may notice water retention. I have found that one to two doses is all you need.

If you implement all the prior steps, you will naturally be optimizing all your hormone levels and will begin leaning out. No peptides required. That's why I created my $3D + 3S + 3M$ protocol, as well as regulating sleep and eliminating stressors.

Fuel Your Muscles

Before introducing exercise, you need to fuel your body with the right fuel, particularly protein, and eating only the amount of carbohydrates that you need for your metabolic rate, as well as your level of activity. You need to supply your body with the right nutrients to build muscle and fuel your mitochondria, as we discussed in chapter 2. To ensure that your microbiome has been optimized, there is an enzyme that is released by bacteria that can cause higher levels of estrogen in the body. That enzyme is called beta-glucuronidase. It cleaves the hydrophilic molecule off estrogen when we're trying to excrete it. We form estrogen and then break it down, form it and then break it down. If you're continually cleaving this molecule, you won't excrete it properly, and your overall circulating levels of estrogen will be higher. This is one cause of estrogen dominance in both men and women. That's why it's crucial to optimize the microbiome in order to have optimal hormone levels.

I've already alluded that there are many toxins in the environment that act as estrogen in the body. Unfortunately, men's testosterone levels have also been found to be 30 percent lower, from 1996 to 2016, according to the

American Urologic Association. Some of this decline is associated with obesity, as well as diabetes, but I suspect that environmental toxins are at play as well.

In a 2010 study, Atrazine-exposed male frogs were demasculinized, or chemically castrated, and completely feminized as adults. This is a shocking statistic, and all the more reason we should look for natural ways when growing our gardens and tending to our lawns. Atrazine is a very commonly used weed killer that can be purchased at many local hardware stores.

Summary

When it comes to exercise, let's recap what we've covered: Exercise regularly; add it into your calendar; make sure your goals are attainable, whether you are at home or traveling; combine cardio, preferably high-intensity interval training with strength training, for a *total* of four to five workouts per week. Ensure adequate protein intake—not only daily, but post-exercise—to maintain and build muscle. Consider consulting with a functional medicine doctor about how to further optimize these steps!

"I never really thought much about those who don't have a purpose, or the impact that would have on one's health, until I retrained in functional medicine. Purpose has actually been found to be so powerful [...] stronger purpose in life was associated with decreased mortality."

Chapter 7

Meaning in Life

The first *M* is "meaning in life," or purpose. This is one of the first questions I ask in my in-depth, twenty-four-page intake form. I recall some years ago watching an *Oprah Winfrey* show in which she was interviewing a psychologist who said the happiest individuals were those living inside of their life's purpose. This made me happy because I was living my life's purpose by practicing medicine. It was my true calling, and I was living in my purpose. I never really thought much about those who don't have a purpose, or the impact that would have on one's health, until I retrained in functional medicine. Purpose has actually been found to be so powerful that, in a 2019 study published by the National Institutes of Health, stronger purpose in life was associated with decreased mortality. This is *huge*.

One of my favorite books on purpose and the ability to survive and overcome is Viktor Frankl's *Man's Search for Meaning.* Viktor Frankl was a psychiatrist who had a huge purpose in life. He was able to endure and survive the German concentration camps during World War II and go on to tell his story. How did he survive? Even barely alive towards the end of his imprisonment, he survived because he had such a strong purpose in life. Read this book, regardless of whether you agree with me or not. It is so powerful.

So, how does one find purpose? Here are my eight top tips:

1. **Develop a growth mindset.** Having a growth mindset has been linked to having a sense of purpose. If you're constantly growing and becoming a better version of yourself, it helps you to identify your purpose. One of the best books on growth mindset was written by Carol Dweck, and it's called *Mindset: The New Psychology of Success*. She contrasts a growth mindset with a fixed mindset and gives you an exact strategy. It's a quick read and not to be missed.

2. **Create a vision statement.** A vision statement makes it easier for you to make decisions aligned with your values; it helps you stay motivated as you work toward your personal goals. I take this one step further: I *love* guided visualization. I love it so much that I have done it most of my adult life. I see things

happening as if they already have, and that's the key to *attracting* positive energy.

3. **Practice gratitude.** Every morning I write down three things for which I'm grateful. After I've finished jotting them down, I oftentimes reach out to people and thank them, or tell them they were on my mind and that I'm grateful for them, or send them an inspirational voice-recorded message. I love voice texts. It's a great pick-me-up, for both me and those around me whom I adore. One of my favorite books on gratitude is *The Last Law of Attraction Book You'll Ever Need to Read* by Andrew Kap. He explores and explains how you have to visualize the life you want as if it *already happened*. This is significantly different than visualizing it from a *wanting* perspective, which attracts negative energy. This book, combined with Dan Sullivan's *The Gap and the Gain*, are must reads. Once I was able to make this shift, all kinds of amazing things happened, and I was also able to overcome a really difficult time last year. It seemed as if everything was going wrong, and I was going to succumb to the stress. But by practicing gratitude and implementing visualization, almost instantaneously I experienced a significant increase in energy. Literally, I walked outside one day, and the

grass seemed greener, the air seemed fresher, and I was never happier. My energy soared. I didn't take a medication or even a single supplement to account for this difference. That is why gratitude is so important for energy, and to feel energized for life!

4. **Give back.** Giving back can enhance your sense of meaning and purpose in life. Look to volunteering in your local community, donate money, or practice random acts of kindness. Pay for the person's coffee behind you in line at the coffee shop, or send a note to someone you've been thinking of who's struggling.

5. **Turn your pain into purpose.** We all face challenges in life. Overcoming them gives us unique strengths and perspectives. Just sharing how we overcame challenges can be helpful to others who may be in the same boat.

6. **Explore new passions.** It is really easy while in the grind of day-to-day living to do nothing that fuels us. Each day feels like a repeat of the day before. Your passion can be your career; maybe it's time for a career change. Or perhaps you should add a new hobby or return to one you let go. A way I've added passion back into my life was first by making Friday Fun Day, only doing things on

Fridays that were fun. Eventually I thought, *Why don't I make every day a fun day, surround myself with like-minded people, and only do things that I love and take time for myself?* It's been a wonderful way to wake up and look forward to each day, further increasing my energy.

7. **Be part of a community.** When you find your purpose, you'll discover that there are others who share similar passions, interests, and values. Joining a community gives you that sense of connection as you work toward a common goal.

8. **Spend time with people who inspire you.** You are the average of the five people with whom you spend the most time! That is why it is so important to be surrounded by like-minded people. It's not only like-minded colleagues in my field with whom I surround myself, but friends as well. I have no less than five dozen girlfriends who would mutually drop everything to help the other out.

All the links to the books referenced above can be found at www.energizedthebook.com/resources. Check them out!

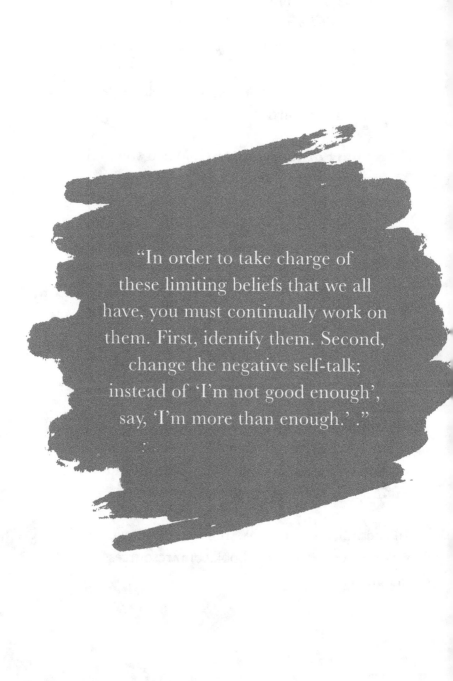

"In order to take charge of
these limiting beliefs that we all
have, you must continually work on
them. First, identify them. Second,
change the negative self-talk;
instead of 'I'm not good enough',
say, 'I'm more than enough.' ."

Chapter 8

Mindset

Mindset is so powerful that I'm giving it its own chapter. I've alluded to how it can help us find purpose in life, but it's much greater than that. It is what keeps people stuck in their own health, so it is crucial to address, especially if your goal is to be an entrepreneur. I've worked on this for forever and a day.

Lissa Rankin writes about how powerful the nocebo effect is in her book *Mind Over Medicine*, meaning if you feel something won't work, it won't. This is in contrast to the placebo effect, in which if you feel it will work, it will. The man who says he can't walk, won't. The man who says he can, will.

Unfortunately, from a young age, we're conditioned to feel certain things that may not be true. All this conditioning usually leads to the limiting belief of "I'm not good enough." Sadly, I'm now seeing this in adolescents who are coming in higher numbers to my office; teenagers were the lowest demographic of patients I'd seen until the last few post-pandemic years.

It is not only things you've been exposed to, but having a fixed mindset that leads to these limiting beliefs. The first person to introduce me to overcoming limiting beliefs was Tony Robbins at his live conference, called "Unleash the Power Within." A girlfriend of mine who was organizing a bunch of health-care practitioners to go asked if I wanted to join them. I had no idea who Tony Robbins was, but because I enjoyed her, and we were like-minded, I said yes. I didn't even think twice, as the tickets were affordable, even the VIP tickets. It fit with my schedule, and I thought, *What the heck? Can't hurt!*

It was one of the best things I've ever done. When I showed up, I was in a stadium filled with almost 40,000 people. These people were chanting, music was blaring, and people were dancing. I texted my husband: Gosh, it feels like a cult, but a good cult!

Tony spent the first day getting you to overcome limiting beliefs. This all led up to the fire walk at 1:00 a.m. at the end of the first day. Yes, I was scared. I was even Googling "people injured at UPW by fire walking." According to Google, no major injuries other than a few minor burns. I was seated next to two amazing women, and together we did the fire walk. We were each other's inspiration. Each night, I came home, and my teenaged son was waiting up to talk to me at 2:00 a.m. We talked seemingly for hours, and then I had to get up and do it again.

A key principle that Tony teaches is rewriting that limiting belief. Take the "I'm not good enough," and turn it into an "I'm more than enough." Maybe you're chanting it, visualizing it, or writing it on a Post-it note. These are all strategies to overcome it. And, for goodness' sake, *let go of anyone who doesn't think you're good enough.* Anyone who makes you feel bad about yourself. Remember what I said? You're the average of the five people with whom you surround yourself.

Another strategy that Tony recommended was, after identifying your beliefs and rewriting them, to take responsibility. The reason why people don't achieve goals is they never take responsibility for their lives. They choose to believe that their circumstances are beyond their control, that things just happen to them. You must believe that life happens *for* you, not *to* you. It's amazing when you make this shift.

The third tip he teaches is to let go of certainty. It's human nature to want certainty, but maintaining this certainty holds you back, and it prevents you from pursuing your dreams or quitting the job that you hate.

A final tip is to change that negative self-talk. That's what I meant when I said rewriting it. Don't believe your own PR (or public relations), or anyone else's for that matter.

Now let's take a look at limiting beliefs and how they relate to health. A study published in 2014 in the *American Journal of Health and Behavior* found that negative beliefs mediate the relationship between depression and health, as well as energy. *What this whole book is about!*

What I would tell any new entrepreneur is to work on mindset first. If you don't work on this, it's the difference between being in the grind and burning out, versus thriving, in regards to how successful you are. I trained as a high-performance coach back in 2019, and I did so because of what I call a "Tale of Two Sisters."

Case Study

Early in my functional medicine career, not even knowing the Dale Bredesen protocol on reversing cognitive decline, I was approached by two women. The first woman was in her early fifties. She was a teacher and had been having extreme difficulty with her memory. By the time I got to the third sentence, she had already forgotten the first two. The impact her memory had was astounding in regards to how it limited her ability to function.

A week later, I saw another slightly older woman who had nearly identical features, spoke similarly, and was almost completely nonfunctional when it came to memory. In fact, she was accompanied by a caregiver and her partner, who had medical power of attorney over her care.

The first sister I was able to work with and take through my 3-D protocol, including my three *S*s and three *M*s. Over the next eighteen months, we were able to successfully restore her memory so that she could begin to thrive.

The second sister was given a diagnosis of "no hope" by a major medical institution and told to go home and die. Okay, maybe not exactly, but you get the picture. I had several hour-long conversations with her medical power of attorney—that is, her partner—and told him the approach that we needed to take. Her care at that point was billed through insurance, but some of my supportive therapies would be out of pocket. Because they had been given no hope, they chose to decline any further care or treatment.

I was absolutely gutted. I didn't have the power to influence them so that they could undertake the steps to at least stop the progression of her decline in memory. I'm almost certain now, almost ten years later, that I could have at least gotten her significant gains.

This is what I call the "Tale of Two Sisters," and it has inspired me to undertake high-performance coaching with Brendon Burchard. One of the tenets he teaches is how to influence, and in this case, I would be using it for the good. Since then, I've actually been coaching high-level entrepreneurs and executives on high performance. If you don't work on your mindset, you'll never succeed in business or in health!

Every time I've gone away and done personal or professional development, I've come back "vibing high." So high that I felt as if I were levitating. My business soared, and that was without doing anything different. Currently, I coach high performers in group settings, as well as one-on-one. In the future, I'll be launching more group programs.

You can find links to these programs at www.energizedthebook.com/resources.

I've oftentimes said the same thing that keeps you from excelling in your health is what will keep you from excelling in your business and in life.

Summary

In order to take charge of these limiting beliefs that we all have, you must continually work on them. First, identify them. Second, change the negative self-talk; instead of "I'm not good enough," say, "I'm more than enough." Take responsibility for your own life. Don't let life happen to you, but for you. Let go of certainty, and take that plunge you've always wanted to take. If you do these simple things on a routine basis, you'll not only succeed in health, but also in your life, and you'll find that your energy soars.

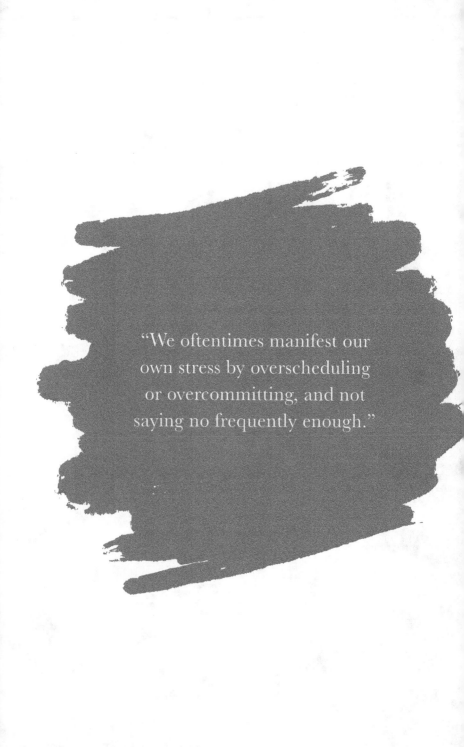

"We oftentimes manifest our own stress by overscheduling or overcommitting, and not saying no frequently enough."

Chapter 9

Time Management

The last step in my nine-step protocol is time management. The formula to be energized and feel fantastic for life is as follows: $3D + 3S + 3M$ = Energized!

We oftentimes manifest our own stress by overscheduling or overcommitting, and not saying no frequently enough. The first thing you need to do to increase your mental energy and ensure that stress doesn't overwhelm and deplete you is to do an inventory of the most important things in your life right now. You need to choose between one and three. One is a good starting point, but if you're a high performer, as I am, you'll almost always have at least three things going on. Really try to limit this to three things so you don't burn out.

Two excellent books have been written on the subject. The first book is *The ONE Thing: The Surprisingly Simple Truth Behind Extraordinary Results* written by Gary Keller and Jay Papasan; it promises that if you focus on one thing, "you'll learn to cut through the clutter, achieve better results in less time, build momentum toward your goal, dial down the stress, overcome that overwhelmed feeling, revive your energy, and stay on track." As a high performer, when I embark on staying up-to-date with functional medicine, I need laser focus. I devote thirty minutes each day, as I prepare breakfast and lunches for my children, to listening to functional medicine lectures. I've done this now, Monday through Friday, for the past decade. Can you imagine the amount of learning this equates to when you are this laser-focused on *one thing*?

What one thing will you be laser-focused on over the next month? I'd love to know. Feel free to share with me by emailing info@simplyhealthinstitute.com. Sharing makes you accountable.

The other book that I recommend to all the high performers I coach is *Essentialism: The Disciplined Pursuit of Less* by Greg McKeown. I devoured this book at the beginning of 2019. I spent several hours creating a plan. In his book, he also says to pick three essential things you'll focus on, and no more. Brendon Burchard teaches the same when it comes to projects: having you set out your goals to align with just three things.

I also love the high-performance strategy of evaluating the opportunity cost. Ask yourself this: Is pursuing this goal making me lose out on other things that are impor-tant? Can I do this activity, or pursue this goal, without costing too much time, energy, effort, resources, and will-power that might be needed somewhere else? This one question alone is what has helped me to decide to say no more often than I say yes.

The next step is to track. Track what you do every waking moment of the day. This will help you identify times of the day that you might be mindlessly scrolling social media. It's astounding how much time can be wasted on social media. I'm not saying it's all bad, but practice mindful social media.

That leads me to the next step. Block out time when you will actually do work towards the three goals you have established. Do not add more goals. More than three can be counterproductive, and you'll burn out. Trust me, I know from personal experience and from coaching hundreds of high performers.

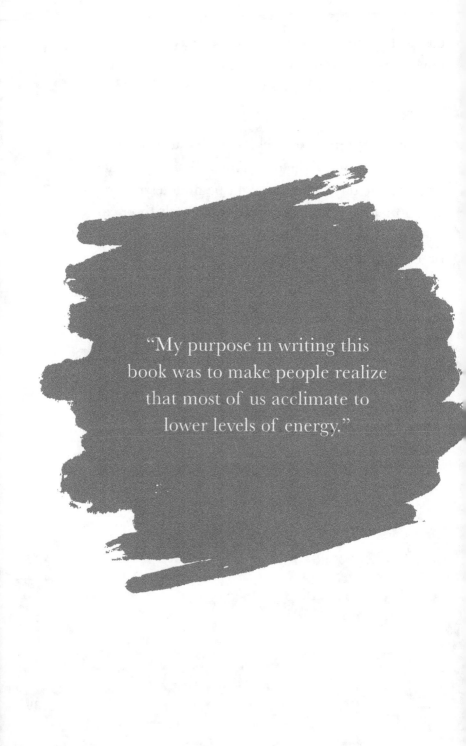

"My purpose in writing this book was to make people realize that most of us acclimate to lower levels of energy."

Chapter 10

Summary and Case Studies

You might be wondering why people would fly across the country, or even from out of the country, *during a pandemic,* just to see me, or why I've been called the Go-To Doctor *for* Doctors. I spent over a decade retraining in functional medicine and absorbing vast amounts of information. I was tutored and mentored by some of the greats, so much so that I was able to craft the $3D + 3S + 3M$ *protocol*, which equals infinite energy!

I thought it would be important to highlight some case studies that would help you understand how I put this protocol into action.

One of the common questions I get asked is: *Will I have enough time?* That's a great question! If you're anything like young Alexandra—a twenty-two-year-old mother of three children, all under the age of five—who, with our support, was walked through the 3-D protocol and was able to eliminate her symptoms of panic attacks and bloating. Her energy got better, her sleep got better, and she became an inspiration to her mother and her husband. She lost ten pounds, and she felt great. That's why she became almost a walking billboard for our clinic: If she could do it, *anyone* could do it, and certainly anyone who doesn't have three children under the age of five!

The other question people ask is: *Will I get results?* No one can guarantee results, but we have been tracking results from our patient base for the past decade, and we consistently see a minimum of 50-percent improvement in symptoms in as little as four weeks. And that's if someone does *modest* amounts of everything. People see far greater gains if they're able to implement even more.

Take for example a nearly seventy-year-old woman who had been struggling to lose weight for a very long time. In the past, she followed any fad diet and lost weight, but with every passing decade, she grew more tired. She had very low energy levels, bloating, and she did not have the energy she needed for herself, let alone to play with her grandchildren. She simply was not going to try yet another diet. By following our 3-D protocol, she was able to get down to a weight she hadn't been since she was in her twenties, she eliminated her bloating, and her energy soared. She saw results she had never seen before.

The next question we get is: *How much does this cost?* Something can either be valuable or expensive. It cannot be both. If you value your health, you must decide how much you are willing to invest in it.

Sadly, I've been part of at least two practices that have failed due to declining insurance reimbursements. After taking insurance for more than seventeen years, I finally decided enough was enough. I did not want to have my patients' care dictated by an algorithm at an insurance company that forced people to jump through hoops, and perhaps not even get the care they need. Let's not even talk about how long it takes these companies to reimburse the typical doctor; you're lucky if you get paid in ninety days, if at all, and it's usually a fraction of what you would bill. Not to mention they certainly don't like paying for extended time with patients.

Our first visit, depending on the level of care you seek, is one and a half hours face-to-face. This does not include the time I spend in advance, meticulously reviewing intake forms and prior labs to start formulating a plan. Once I meet with you, this plan gets finalized because we *collaborate* on the next steps that you are going to take. We also have Executive Edge clients who are high performers seeking to not only eliminate symptoms, but gain knowledge about anti-aging and longevity measures. We spend two hours face-to-face, and with the time spent on the back end, at checkout, and finalizing notes and coordinating care, it's a total of almost four hours. After the labs are back, I spend as much time as needed with my patients to discuss their results. Before these visits? You guessed it; I'm reviewing a patient's chart so we can determine what worked, what didn't work, as well as doing a deep dive into all their labs. This includes comparing their results to any prior labs that we had run so I never miss a beat. This fits in with our three values at Simply Health Institute for providing a high level of service, and it is part of why I feel that we get better results than many other functional medicine doctors.

We value complete transparency, which is why we perform discovery calls. We want people who *want* the services we offer. We want people who are mutually respectful and will work collaboratively with us—those who will take a full mind/body approach and those who will address stored, underlying trauma. And, lastly, we just want to have fun. We always practice from a high level of integrity, whether it's recommending a lab or a supplement supplier. Transparency, integrity, and a high level of service—that's what we're all about. I would say, without a shadow of a doubt, to date, this practice is 100 percent full of the most wonderful people you could ever imagine being able to serve.

Let's talk about one of my favorite patients. She is a thirty-eight-year-old woman who had significant joint pain in her hands and feet. Very similar to her younger sister, who was diagnosed with lupus at the age of eighteen, this patient reported the following: She went and saw a rheumatologist who spoke to her for all of two minutes, gave her a lab order, and then a few weeks later sent her a message in the patient portal saying her labs were normal, that she didn't have lupus, and to come back if she felt worse.

That was the wrong answer. Clinically, she was trending towards and exhibiting signs of acute, full-blown lupus. It was causing low energy and severe symptoms that almost made her quit her job. Within two short weeks, she did everything and was 70 percent better. Yes, she was a real go-getter and wanted to do everything I had in my army of tools to get better. By six weeks, she was 90 percent better, and by three months, she felt as if she had never even had lupus. She went on to exercise regularly and implement stress-modification techniques. These were techniques that I not only teach, but emphasize need to be used *every day* for prolonged resiliency. She reduced her hours at work for a while, and when she resumed full-time work and was inevitably faced with the same stressors that would have thrown her under the bus before, she did *not* get thrown under the bus, she did *not* feel burnout, and she did *not* have a flare-up of symptoms.

She recently wrote to us and said she is absolutely thrilled at the level of energy she has. Before, she could not have imagined running three miles, let alone running, training, and completing a marathon. She's reengaging our services to ensure that she remains well.

Visits to the functional medicine doctor should be no different than visits to your dentist. If you don't go to your dentist for many years, you can't expect to have healthy teeth. It's the same in traditional medicine and functional medicine. Don't wait for your tests and symptoms to worsen or become so far gone that your condition is difficult to control and treat.

I have many cases in which I have completely changed people's lives. One young entrepreneur, James, came to me in his early thirties. He had been disabled from work for a full two years. He was lucky in the respect that he had established a successful business and was able to work limited hours throughout the week to be able to support himself. However, he was unlucky because he felt as if his whole life had been stolen. He had even come up with a plan to commit assisted suicide. He had all his friends and family on board.

Can you imagine? He was only thirty! He had fallen in love and gotten engaged to a young woman, but he couldn't even stand long enough to take engagement photos. I met with him first virtually because he was too unwell to fly. Then he saw me in my office one month later. After implementing changes I had advised him to make, he had 90-percent improvement in his fatigue only four weeks later! He was almost fully back to normal and functional. While we still had work to do, these were astonishing results. He and his fiancée invited us out to dinner, and we accepted, which I don't often do, but I wanted to oblige him. They were just the loveliest couple.

A month later, they invited us to their wedding. At his wedding, he wore a tie clip that said, "I'm healthy," because all he could think about when he was unwell, which was on and off for most of his life, but particularly these past two years, was *getting healthy*. That was the only goal he had. I will never forget how humbled I felt when I was the first person he toasted for giving him his life back. I was so grateful to have been able to serve him and to see him get back to working on his business, to see him acquire another business, and to see him have his first child, who's now just over a year old. None of these things would have been possible if he had continued to feel so unwell.

It is James's story and the story of so many others like him that inspire me to keep going—to keep learning, to listen to lectures, not only while I make breakfast and lunches in the morning, but now even in the shower, using a waterproof speaker. I know that seems nerdy, but I am so passionate about health and wellness, particularly functional medicine and longevity, that I can't get enough! It's similar to drinking from a fire hose.

There was another young lady who came to me at twenty-eight years old. She saw me late summer 2020. She was about to return to school to complete her PhD. She had only one quarter left, but she feared that she didn't have enough energy to finish, which was also wearing on her emotional energy. She felt pressure to complete schooling in the next three months, something she had worked so hard to do. By the time we had taken her through the 3-D protocol, she was astounded at the energy she had and how all her symptoms had resolved. She went from being weak, sick, and tired, getting chronic recurring infections that lasted for weeks, to a vibrant, healthy young lady who graduated with her PhD on time. She also went on to say that, prior to seeing me, she could not even walk a full city block. But, a year later, she had run a marathon and had run it well!

I had another woman who came to me also very sick and tired. She was in her late sixties and had developed severe right upper-quadrant pain. They had assumed it was her gallbladder, despite an ultrasound that was only mildly abnormal. In the process, she had her gallbladder removed, which only served to worsen her pain. She got so sick that she was losing weight. She was intolerant of many foods, and the pain was worse. I saw her for her first consultation and noticed a very large, sausage-shaped mass on her thyroid. It was seven centimeters. That couldn't have grown overnight, so how did this get missed?

Unfortunately for her, it was thyroid cancer, which had nothing to do with her abdominal pain, and probably only modestly contributed to her fatigue. But, fortunately for her, it was slow-growing, and she only needed to have her thyroid gland removed in order for her to have resolution of this cancer. After we walked her through our 3-D protocol, she had complete resolution of her abdominal pain, regained her energy, and started tolerating more and more foods.

Another woman came to me who was a stay-at-home mom and homeschooled her children. She supported her husband in his business and was well known in her community. She had experienced brain fog and fatigue for a decade. That's right—a *decade*. When we did her discovery call, I gave some recommendations that she could implement prior to coming to see me because we had a two-month waiting list at that point. I quickly identified that she likely had limbic-system dysfunction.

The limbic system is like the security system for our house; it should only alarm when there's a true invader. But when you're subjected to toxins—in her case it was an environmental toxin—her limbic system alarmed all the time. When that occurs, you're not only in fight-or-flight all the time, but every attempt to make these people better can actually make them worse. Even the simplest of supplements or medications can make them sicker. Things need to be started slower and advanced slower than in the ordinary patient.

I'd given her a few recommendations, and she implemented them. However, a couple of weeks later, we got a not-so-nice email, and it was clear that she was distressed. She wanted to know how I could expect anyone to implement this level of retraining when they felt so unwell? Well, she persisted, and at the six-week mark, she said she had full resolution of her brain fog and wanted to cancel her appointment. I had a short conversation with her and explained we hadn't figured out what exactly triggered all these symptoms, and that she'd only regress.

She came in, and we made her better and better. She went from almost dysfunctional and not exercising, to fully functional and walking an hour every single day. She soon went on to send us many of her friends in the community, including a young woman who suffered from severe migraines.

When this young woman came in, her second daughter was just four months old. She was really struggling to be a good mom because her headaches were so debilitating. We worked with her to reduce her headaches down to almost none, and at the end of the 3-D protocol, she went on to get pregnant, saying it was the best pregnancy she'd had, and she was full of energy. She ended up delivering a vibrant, robust, happy baby boy.

Another gentleman was not even forty years old when he came to me. He was working full time as a medical doctor. He'd started a medical business in another state, which necessitated that he travel all the time. He admitted he wasn't eating as well as he should. He wasn't exercising as he wanted to, and the wear and tear of travel and level of stress was getting to him. His energy had plummeted, and his testosterone levels were in the gutter.

Unfortunately for him, he had seen another doctor in the area who put him on testosterone. Testosterone is not indicated for men under the age of forty-five or so. In addition, that doctor was not monitoring him, nor did he take a good history from this patient. If he had, he would have learned that this young man's father had developed breast cancer. This would have made any doctor, who was familiar with hormones and how they were broken down in the body, take pause and measure levels before, during, and after treatment with testosterone. It's a clinical sign that very likely this man's father converted testosterone more readily to estrogen, and probably this patient did as well.

Again, unfortunately, for him while his energy might have improved a little, the testosterone quickly converted to estrogen, and he developed "man boobs", or gynecomastia, which is a very undesirable effect if you're a man. Fortunately, he was able to get on an aromatase inhibitor to block that conversion of testosterone to estrogen, and he went off the testosterone as a result. He also implemented a healthier diet and better lifestyle choices. As we walked him through the 3-D protocol, his testosterone levels normalized with gentle supplementation, and his energy resumed.

In my earlier years, I had three women come to me from the same company. Sadly, they were all high-level executives who had retired in their early fifties, which was fifteen years earlier than they had planned. All three were fatigued and burned out with a variety of symptoms. The first woman, Laurie, was fatigued, her skin was breaking out, she had bloating, and she didn't sleep well. She'd developed an autoimmune disease called Graves, or hyperthyroidism, which is an autoimmune disease. I took her through my 3-D protocol, and she had complete resolution of her symptoms. She just recently has gone on to launch her own business, on her own terms, so that she can live her life in balance. The second patient from this company, Silvana, came to me with fatigue and a tremor. The same thing happened; we walked her through the 3-D protocol, and her tremor disappeared, her fatigue resolved, and she felt better than ever. Typically, when I hear of a tremor, I think of toxin exposure, and this was one of her main issues. She went on to feel so good that she sent me her brother and her nearly ninety-year-old father, who recovered quickly. I even developed a hashtag in his honor: #belikefrank.

Frank came to see me at eighty-nine years of age, and until recently he had exhibited no medical issues. Frank developed bladder cancer and needed surgery as part of the treatment protocol. After that surgery, he ended up feeling extremely fatigued. Within one month of implementing my 3-D protocol, his energy soared, and I very rarely saw him (which was a good thing!). What did Frank do that many of my other patients didn't? He was Italian and ate all whole foods. He grew most of his own vegetables, and if he ate any animal protein, it was fish. He surrounded himself with friends and community; he was physically active, both at the gym and outside in his garden. He did everything right. The only mistake I was able to pinpoint was that he didn't filter his water, and, yep, you guessed it—toxins in water can contribute to bladder cancer.

Let's take a look at this issue closer. Why is it that some people live longer and live well, while others either die an early death or suffer in their later years? When I was first in practice, my under-eighty-year-old patients seemed vibrant, but as time went on, they seemed less and less so. For one year, I worked doing Medicare physicals for senior citizens in their homes, and there was a distinct difference between the eighty-plus-year-old patients who were vibrant and full of vitality, and those who were not. What was the difference? Here's what I observed: The healthier seniors almost always had partners. They had a sense of purpose, usually in their church, or they were an active part of a tight-knit community. They ate mostly whole foods, and they exercised, with many of them belonging to Silver Sneakers, which is a reduced-rate program at the gym. They all were on some form of gentle supplementation, with most of them taking a multivitamin, fish oil, and vitamin D, which is what I recommend all my patients take at a bare minimum, although I also add in a probiotic and magnesium in most instances.

I will be including a bonus chapter on longevity (to those who buy during the launch periods!), with a deep dive into utilizing diet plus lifestyle, along with peptides for anti-aging purposes, to ensure you can live long, well.

Remember when I said that some patients who came to see me thought they felt well, but then at the end of their time working with me, they ALL said they didn't realize they could feel this fantastic? That is my goal for you!

If you like this book, could you do me a favor? Share this book with a loved one. And even better yet, leave me a five-star review on Amazon. Let's spread the word!

My purpose in writing this book was to make people realize that most of us acclimate to lower levels of energy. This lower level of energy starts because most people are born deficient in a handful of vitamins and minerals. These vitamins and minerals get depleted over time, after exposure to chronic stressors. Then, after years of exposure to the usual toxins, the toxins not only further deplete nutrients, but they also take out the mitochondria, which are not protected in regard to their DNA, as the rest of our DNA is. So, not only was the goal to highlight the fact that most people acclimate to a lower level of energy, but to provide valuable tools to help people reclaim the energy of their youth.

I suffered from low energy for almost three decades. I thought I was going to leave my children motherless, and I almost was unable to actualize my three dreams: becoming a doctor, having my own family, and owning my own practice in which I would attempt to cure as many people as I could.

I hope this book will help prevent needless suffering in millions in the years to come. Thank you for reading.

To Simply Health,

With love,

Dr. Rajka

Acknowledgments

First and foremost, I want to thank you, the reader! Without you, there would not be a book. So thank you!

There are so many people who supported me along the way; without this support, I wouldn't have become the physician that I am today. I want to ensure I take the time to acknowledge each and every one of you, including family, friends, colleagues, my team and prior staff, mentors, and teachers, as well as patients. To my two biggest cheerleaders: my mom and sister. My mom just showed up! She was there to witness every milestone, including crossing the finish line of my first marathon (making my sister drive her two hours to see me finish!), serving as our nanny for one year when ours fell through, and flying to every city we lived in from Seattle to Chicago, to Qatar, and to Boston. She even celebrated New Year's Eve with us in Kelowna, Canada, although she didn't ski. She worked three jobs to help move our family out of the inner city of Cleveland and to pay for my two siblings and me to attend college. She even covered the first hour of my 7:00 a.m. laundry shift at the nursing home, allowing me an extra hour of sleep as my waitressing job ended at 2:30 a.m. This was before her job began at 8:00 a.m. She nicknamed me first Rocky and then Chu Chu, and most recently Rocko.

My sister, Bonnie Wolff, aka Chi Chi, is wise beyond her years. She's the baby whisperer, always there with a compassionate ear. We have spent hours supporting each other. You are more than enough and one of the best mamas I know.

To my father, who never doubted my dream of becoming a doctor and always believed in my capabilities. When I asked him to teach me to paint and repair things, he said, "You don't need to know how to do these things! You will always have me!" Little did either of us know that he would pass away when I was thirty years of age. I wish I had known then what I know now… I feel I could have saved him from an early death.

Thankfully, my brother stepped in, as is customary in the Serbian culture. From buying me an interview outfit for both medical school and residency, to even paying for some of my medical school (something I only learned in my fifties!), to walking me down the aisle (I was so honored). Your text filled with kind words after I hit best-seller status for this book is something I will never forget. You are the big brother every sister should have.

Thank you to Kerry, my soulmate, who has forever and a day said, "I'm a believer." So many adventures: two children, two continents, multiple cities and jobs, and one dog. It has been a fabulous ride. I love you with all my heart.

Liam, you are my gentle giant, now towering over me and your dad at over six feet. I love how our relationship has grown now that you are an adult, to mentor and mentee and no longer parent and child. I can already see all the great things you will do with your life. I love your mind—so bright—your kind heart, and your efficient ways.

Liv, I am prouder of you than you will ever know. I love how you are kind to all your peers, how you silently lead, how you are proud of your work, and how you leave each place better and more joyful than you found it. I see you excelling in whatever you choose to do in the future. The dog does really love you more than me.

To my extended family: the Milanovics, Grujics, Stevanovics, Wolffs, and Corsettis. I am in awe of your support when my book launched. You were all the first to buy. Thank you for all the fun times: countless family dinners, outings, and vacations. May we have many more. It really has been like *Four Weddings and a Funeral* and *My Big Fat Greek Wedding* all rolled into one.

To my favorite mentor, Dr. Skully! You were a fav for so many of us. You saved me from throwing in the towel on a career that I have grown to fall in love with again.

To Ed Levitan, my first mentor in functional medicine. I am deeply grateful to have been mentored on every patient every day for three months. It allowed me to expedite my learning of functional medicine and has allowed me impact even more lives!

Dr. Neil Nathan, you taught me that healing the seemingly incurable was possible. I love the community of heart-centered practitioners you have created. It is one of the only groups in which I have never felt judged.

Sachin Patel, you saved me from giving up on a practice that was barely profitable, teaching me strategies to make it soar and teaching me to believe in myself even more.

JJ Virgin, I love that you empower, inspire, and lift up so many others. The tide really does raise all boats! I have thoroughly appreciated all your support and guidance, especially as the road got bumpy. You have become like a sister. Keep shining your bright light.

Nat Kringoudis, your strategy sessions have made me think outside of the box. You are a champion of women, both in health and entrepreneurship. Your ideas our ingenious.

To my team—Julie Kerr and Lauren Rafferty Svitak—I don't know what I would do without you ladies. You truly have embraced the vision and mission of providing a high level of service. I am grateful for your support, especially when I go out of town to promote the book, speak on news stations, and attend conferences.

I have been fortunate to have worked with some amazing support staff through the years; it would be difficult to name you all. Thank you to each and every one of you.

I will always fondly remember my first nurse, Christine Dunbar, who was the one to give the practical advice to so many moms and allowed my patients' voices to be heard.

I have long been a champion of empowering women and am blessed to have over fifty (yes, fifty!) women whom I can call my friend and know that if I called upon you, you would just show up to support me. This theme of a community of women has been a common thread in my life and is what makes me thrive. I am excited to soon be launching my women's community—Radiantly SHE—that will empower women to live long, well, and in turn have them empower their own tribes to do the same. I will acknowledge these women next.

To my three best friends: Achina, Brenda, and Christina. You each came into my life nearly a decade apart. Brenda, we spent our thirties painting the town red in Seattle, sharing dreams and aspirations during our formative years. So many road trips and adventures. I cherish our friendship.

Christina, you gave me hope when I returned to Qatar after fully expecting to be back in the USA for good. Your vision and mission in empowering women and launching

Qatar Professional Women's Network was just the inspiration I needed. I stepped into your shoes for one event when you were away and was humbled at the respect you commanded from those 2,000 women. I am further humbled by your support this past decade. I love you to pieces!

Achina, all it took was one conversation after work, and we were fast friends as if we had known each other for years. I enjoyed all our dinners in our home when Kerry was away. You not only kept things lighthearted and fun, but were a source of support during the many hiccups that ensued during Kerry's absence. I love how you have loved my kids! You have a beautiful mind and are hands down one of the best physicians I know. Your patients are lucky to have you. Our couple's trip to Paris, filled with belly laughs, was so memorable and much needed.

To my Buckeye Girls: Julie Manchester, Dr. Monica Lutz, Dr. Melissa Young-Szalay, Dr. Jennifer Graygar, and Jodi Barnum Lohrey. I look forward to our yearly girls' trips. We've shared an incredible journey with its highs and lows in this adventure called life. I'd drop everything to support each of you, and I know you'd do the same for me.

To my Hot Crayons: Dr. Achina Stein, Dr. Ana Marie Temple, Dr. Amie Hornaman, Dr. Betty Murray, Sarah Clark, Jess Mc Naughton, Dr. Tabatha Barber, Dr. Lisa Oslewieski, Dr. Aimee Apigian, Kim West, and Jackie Bowker. I am so grateful to have found you through Mindshare Mastermind and love how supportive we have grown of each other the past two years, from our daily texts to our monthly mastermind meetings. I would not have made it this far without you all.

To my very first best friend, Maria Vovos, my half-Serbian sister. Our childhood summers have a special place in my heart: riding our bikes until the sun went down, drinking Kool-Aid until our bellies hurt, playing softball, and warding off the bully girls.

To my middle school and high school girlfriends: Angela Musial, Michelle Carbone, and Beth Germaine Rodeo. Mish, who would've thought that our shared vanity about not taking swimming during the school year would spark a lifelong bond? The pandemic and the time following have brought us closer than ever before.

To my college girlfriends: Shelly Lenz, my study buddy and a woman I have always admired. Amy Hay Schwab, it was so fun being Rho Chis together. I have loved watching your girls grow up. Jessica Bittence, I couldn't imagine a better friend with whom to go through residency.

Dr. Brenda Flake, you are a class act. I looked up to you and was happy to have you as a role model when I started in private practice. I have so enjoyed getting together with you over the years, although it is not frequent enough.

Marcy Cox, I so enjoyed our Doha Daze, giving each other Keratin treatments at home, dishing about life, health, and wellness. You are a gem.

To my favorite group of former women colleagues in Boston: Achina Stein, Patti Zub, Sophia DaRosa, Lisa Vasile, Janice Pegels, Ziesl Mayaan, Nicole Pichette, Kari Emsbo, Bev Wedda, Noelle Lee, Kathleen Dichiara, and Julianne Goicoechea. Grateful that Visions Healthcare brought us together.

Monica Donath, Shweta Kamal, Maggie Homolka, Louise Porter, and Carla Bausch: You are my local peeps, always fun, although our busy lives don't allow nearly enough time for socializing. Monica, I love how our relationship has blossomed from patient to friend and how you have been like an auntie to our children. We love you Monica!

To my local functional medicine dynamite group of women practitioners: Dr. Dina Pavilonis, Joya Van der Laan, Dr. Catherine Johnson, Dr. Aleesha Fisher, Dr. Anju Usman, and Dr. Madiha Saeed. Our busy lives, practices, and families don't allow for nearly enough time with any of you. Madiha, I'm deeply thankful for your support during my mom's visit. Her trip, likely her last due to her health, was possible because of you. I'll always treasure the three months we had with her. Plus, our laughter during the last Mindshare Summit is unforgettable.

To all the other women colleagues scattered across the world: Dr. Kat Toups, you are the biggest "go-giver" I know. I will never forget celebrating each of us scoring in the top quartile on the IFM certification exam (the hardest exam I have ever taken). Your knowledge amazes me. Dr. Cammy Benton, a true champion of natural medicine, you are my hero, more courageous than I could ever be, especially during the pandemic.

To my fellow Perfect Practice coaches—Dr. Liana Rodriguez, Natalie Morse, and Miranda Summer: You all take things to the next level. It has been a privilege to grow as a coach with all of you.

To Dr. Betsy Greenleaf, Dr. Elisa Song, Dr. Krista Burns, Dr. Deb Matthew, and Claudia Muehlenweg—my fellow Mindshare Masterminders: You all inspire me, and I have so enjoyed your support.

While I have always cherished my female friends, I would be amiss if I didn't mention some of my "brothers." My Everett Family Practice Center colleagues: Dr. Tom Koewler, the late Dr. Arthur Grossman (you were taken from us too soon!), Dr. Bruce Kennedy (a class act—I will never forget how everyone thought we were a couple when you took me to see *Madame Butterfly!*), and Dr. Bud Wagner (I had big shoes to fill when you retired!).

To my Perfect Practice brothers, Dr. David Bennett and Dr. Buddy Touchinsky: You are upstanding doctors, husbands, and fathers, and I am lucky to call you brothers! I have so enjoyed coaching with you and watching you grow into your highest selves.

Dr. Pedro Gonzalez, I have so enjoyed sharing peptide cases with you.

To my editor, Nicole Soule-Roberts: Your skills in making my words shine are priceless. Thank you!

And to my publisher, Lisa M. Umina, and her team at Halo Publishing: So grateful to you for making this experience seamless and enjoyable.

A special thank-you to Dr. Jose Colon who not only introduced me to Lisa, but who spent several hours helping me support a sick family member!

The utmost gratitude is reserved for my patients across the globe: from Columbus, Ohio; to Everett, Washington; to Chicago, Illinois; to Boston, Massachusetts; and to Qatar. You make me be a better doctor by asking me questions that keep me on my toes and inspire me to learn more. My very first practice, Everett Family Practice Center, will always carry a special place in my heart. It truly was a place like *Cheers*, where everyone knew your name! I am grateful that my current practice, Simply Health Institute, allows me to make the biggest difference and to reverse the seemingly irreversible.

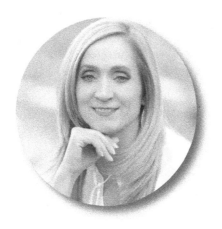

About the Author

D r. Rajka Milanovic Galbraith is a revered triple-board-certified doctor in family medicine, integrative medicine, and functional medicine. After battling nearly three decades of debilitating fatigue herself, she emerged triumphant, not only restoring her own energy, but also revitalizing the lives of thousands of others. Her unparalleled expertise has earned her the nickname the Energizer Bunny, and has made her the go-to doctor among physicians. She sees patients in her clinic, Simply Health Institute, outside of Chicago and does high-performance coaching of entrepreneurs.

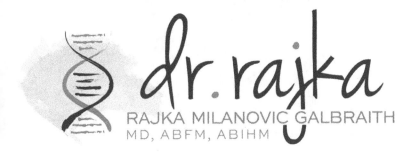

RAJKA MILANOVIC GALBRAITH
MD, ABFM, ABIHM

About the Dr. Rajka Brand

D r Rajka's values are 2 fold: Transparency, high integrity and providing a high level of service. The ultimate goal is to prevent needless suffering AND empower people to their highest state of energy and health so they may empower their tribes: family, friends and colleagues.

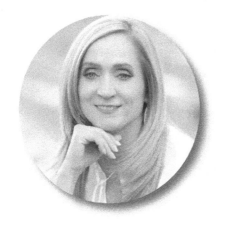

Let's Connect

Find out more about Rajka Milanovic Galbraith, MD
at the following links!

www.drrajka.com

Email: info@simplyhealthinstitute.com

IG: @drrajka

FB: www.facebook.com/drrajka

YouTube:www.youtube.com/channel/
UC9BNmgntX3scI6tKpsMmfpQ

Printed in the USA
CPSIA information can be obtained
at www.ICGtesting.com
CBHW072303070924
14239CB00003B/23

9 781637 654842